Lymphedema

Ordering

Trade bookstores in the U.S. and Canada please contact:
Publishers Group West
1700 Fourth Street, Berkeley CA 94710
Phone: (800) 788-3123   Fax: (510) 528-3444

Hunter House books are available at bulk discounts for textbook course adoptions; to qualifying community, healthcare, and government organizations; and for special promotions and fundraising. For details please contact:

Special Sales Department
Hunter House Inc., PO Box 2914, Alameda CA 94501-0914
Tel. (510) 865-5282   Fax (510) 865-4295
e-mail: ordering@hunterhouse.com

Individuals can order our books from most bookstores or by calling toll-free:
1-800-266-5592

Lymphedema

A
Breast Cancer Patient's Guide to Prevention and Healing

by Jeannie Burt & Gwen White, P.T.

Hunter House
PUBLISHERS

Hunter House Inc., Publishers
P.O. Box 2914
Alameda CA 94501-0914

Library of Congress Cataloging-in-Publication Data

Burt, Jeannie.
Lymphedema : a breast cancer patient's guide to prevention and healing / by Jeannie Burt and Gwen White. – 1st ed.
p. cm
ISBN 0-89793-265-X (cloth). — ISBN 0-89793-264-1 (paper)
1. Lymphedema. 2. Breast—Cancer—Treatment—Complications.
I. White, Gwen, P.T. II. Title.
RC646.3.B87 1999
616.4'2—dc21   99-32471
CIP

Project Credits
Cover Design: Kathy Warinner   Book Design & Production: Hunter House
Copy Editor: Rosana Francescato   Developmental Editor: Priscilla Stuckey
Proofreader: Lee Rappold   Indexer: Kathy Talley-Jones
Acquisitions Coordinator: Jeanne Brondino
Project Editors: Kiran Rana, Jennifer Rader
Production Director: Virginia Fontana   Illustrations: Kathy Albert
Publicity Director: Marisa Spatafore   Special Sales Manager: Sarah Kulin
Publisher's Assistant and Website Coordinator: Georgia Moseley
Customer Support: Christina Sverdrup, Joel Irons
Order Fulfillment: A & A Quality Shipping Services
Publisher: Kiran S. Rana

Printed and bound by Publishers Press, Salt Lake City, Utah
Manufactured in the United States of America

9 8 7 6 5 4 3 2 1   First Edition   99 00 01 02 03

Table of Contents

The numbers in superscript in the text refer to endnotes
organized by chapter and starting on page 188.

Foreword

I am delighted to be asked to write a foreword to this book.

Lymphedema has long been a largely ignored complication following cancer. Some people are simply born with lymphatic insufficiency and may have had the condition for many years. In most cases, patients have been told lymphedema is something they just have to live with and that nothing can be done for them. This is simply not true.

As our knowledge has grown over the years, treatment procedures have greatly improved, and so has our understanding of the disease. Diagnostic techniques have been greatly developed, and there is an increased awareness on the part of both the medical profession and the public in general.

Early diagnosis and an immediate treatment course with carfully individualized education on self-management is essential. Maintaining this self-care will lead to further reduction, and will take only a short time on a daily basis. This means that the focus of the patient's life will not be on her lymphedema, but on what she can achieve and enjoy without further complications. With compliance and self-care, a positive outcome, in terms of both self-esteem and well-being, lies in the patient's own hands.

Patient support groups now exist worldwide. The Lymphoedema Association of Australia (L.A.A.) was one of the first to be formed in 1982, and our first large patient meeting was held in Adelaide, Australia, at the International Society of Lymphology congress in 1985. Knowledge regarding patient care and treatment has spread to most countries of the world. Home pages on the Internet are providing valuable rescue material and contact data. But this information is not yet available to everyone, which is why a book like this is so useful.

This is an important publication from a number of points of view.

First, it gives clear information on what lymphedema is and why it occurs. Second, it describes treatment procedures to suit a range of needs and emphasizes that lymphedema can be treated successfully. Of even more value, it gives patients hope for their future. They will know on reading this that they are not alone and that there are many avenues of help and support available.

I congratulate the authors for their persistence in this project and on a work well done. I wish it every success. I am sure that it will be extremely useful to people with lymphedema and give them hope and courage to manage their condition better. It must not rule their lives; with care and understanding of their condition, people with lymphedema can live a full life.

JUDITH R. CASLEY-SMITH, M.D.
Malvern, Australia
April 1999

Acknowledgments

Bringing a book like this to fruition would not be possible without the efforts and guidance of many people, and we wish to thank everyone who helped make this book a reality. We are especially grateful for the support, encouragement, and expertise of Drs. Stephen Chandler, James Schwarz, Michael Goldman, Judith R. Casley-Smith, and Robert Lerner. We owe a debt of gratitude to the professionalism and vision of Saskia R. J. Thiadens, R.N., Ruth Bach, M.Ed., L.P.C., Izetta Smith, M.A., and Vicki Romm, L.C.S.W.

We also want to thank Joan Weddle, Shirley Schreiner, Kathryn Tierney, Nancy Espinoza, R.N., Barbara Henarie, Dolf Dolson, Julene Fox, Nancy Friedemann, R.N., and Vera Wheeler, R.N., for the gifts of their time and experience. Without their generosity this book would not have been possible.

Important Note

The material in this book is intended to provide a review of information regarding lymphedema and its treatment. Every effort has been made to provide accurate and dependable information. The contents of this book have been compiled through professional research and in consultation with medical professionals. However, health care professionals have differing opinions and advances in medical and scientific research are made very quickly, so some of the information may become outdated.

Therefore, the publisher, authors, editors, and any professionals quoted in the book cannot be held responsible for any error, omission, or dated material. The authors and publisher assume no responsibility for any outcome of applying the information in this book in a program of self-care or under the care of a licensed practitioner. If you have questions about the application of the information described in this book, consult a qualified health care professional.

Preface

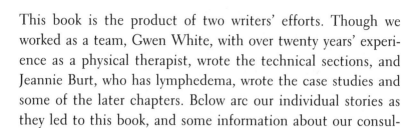

This book is the product of two writers' efforts. Though we worked as a team, Gwen White, with over twenty years' experience as a physical therapist, wrote the technical sections, and Jeannie Burt, who has lymphedema, wrote the case studies and some of the later chapters. Below are our individual stories as they led to this book, and some information about our consultants on the project.

We hope you will find this book both informative and comforting. We also hope it will give you a means to find help for your lymphedema so you can deal with it and release whatever hold it has on your life. Read on. There is help, and with help there is hope.

Jeannie Burt's Story

I know about lymphedema. I have had it since May of 1997, just weeks after I finished chemotherapy and radiation for breast cancer.

The swelling was gradual at first, and I thought it would go away. Then it just ballooned one hot, humid weekend after I transplanted a patch of overgrown daisies. My whole arm looked like it was being smothered in lumpy white flesh. My shoulder began to ache. My elbow became bloated and fiery hot.

On Monday, I tried to call my oncologist. He was out, the receptionist said, gone for a week. A week! A lifetime!

I tried to tell myself I could wait for my doctor, that everything would be okay. But, in truth, I started to panic. At night I couldn't sleep. My imagination kicked in in a way it hadn't since I was a child conjuring demons. How much more lopsided and huge would I get before I talked to my doctor? I'd hold up my arm and shake it. I felt totally out of control. The bed sheets would knot around me as I squeezed my elbow and did some exercises with my hand. And, by morning, my arm would still be swollen.

During the day, I was turning into a witch consumed with worry. My parents called from their farm three hundred miles away. I told them about the swelling, then flew into a tirade when they didn't give it the concern I thought they should have. My husband was worried and puzzled and looked as though he felt helpless himself. He was beginning to hold my hand and just let me rant. No one seemed to understand why, after all I'd gone through with cancer, *this* was bothering me so much. But it was.

I couldn't wait. I had to do something, to take some kind of action. I decided to find out as much as I could before my doctor came back. I dug around in the old papers my cancer clinic had given me when I was told I had cancer. There was a bunch of stuff: pages on chemo drugs, a whole booklet on arranging hats and scarves on a head with no hair, reams of disclaimers, instructions on what not to eat before surgery. Yet there was just one measly line mentioning possible swelling, and it gave the swelling a name: lymphedema. When my husband came home that day after work, I waved that sheet of paper in his face and screamed, "At least I have a name for it!"

I went to the library. I'd be exaggerating if I said the library had nothing on lymphedema. Two books on breast cancer mentioned it: a total of three paragraphs. Both books said there wasn't much to do about it.

I felt totally lost, hopeless. Self-pity is not normally a big emotion for me. Well, let me tell you, I was wallowing in it.

My oncologist finally got back from his trip. His voice was gentle on the phone, as if he realized how troubled I was. He told me about Gwen and assured me there were new techniques for dealing with lymphedema. I have since come to realize how lucky I was that my doctor knew about lymphedema and knew how to get me help. Most doctors, it seems, still don't know about the help that is available.

My course of therapy began. Gwen not only treated my lymphedema but also instructed me in helping myself. Knowing what to do gave me back power and control. And she didn't stop with simply helping me, but willingly took time from her tremendously busy life to co-write this book so others might not feel at such an awful loss as I once did.

This book holds the information I craved so long ago.

My life now is back where I want it to be. I don't think a stranger would know I ever had an episode of lymphedema. It took effort to get the swelling down, and it took patience, but it worked. I know I will always be vulnerable to another episode, so I'm careful and still follow Gwen's teaching. It's not a bad outcome.

If you have lymphedema, or are just concerned about its potential, please read on. If someone—your doctor, your nurse, anyone—tells you there is nothing to do about lymphedema, don't believe them. There's plenty you can do, my friend. The information in this book should help you.

Gwen White's Story

I clearly recall the first time (and it doesn't seem that long ago) I ever heard the term *manual lymph drainage*. I had been a physical therapist for over twenty-two years, specializing in work with patients with head and facial pain in a Temporomandibular Disorders Clinic. I had another area I loved working in—that of health education. I was involved in facilitating and teaching different health education programs. My third and actually most important job in my life is that of being a mother to three children, who were all under eleven years old at that time.

One day at a staff meeting in 1996, my boss said that the Oncology Department in our clinic (and organization) was pressuring him to have someone provide this new treatment—lymphatic massage—for patients with lymphedema. Evidently, some well-informed patients had been insisting on this "new" treatment. My boss asked for someone to volunteer to be involved with the program. My cup felt pretty full at the time (in fact, at times it seemed to runneth over), and volunteering crossed my mind for only a second, as I wondered what this treatment was.

No one volunteered. Then my boss said that whoever volunteered would be going down to Anaheim to the Hyatt Regency the following week for a four-day training in lymphedema management for breast cancer patients with Linda Miller, P.T. I quickly mentally reviewed my schedule, my kids' schedules, and my husband's schedule and decided that I could potentially arrange to go. My hand went up as I thought I could really use a break from the regular schedule—and four days at the Hyatt Regency sounded wonderful, whatever this lymphatic massage stuff was.

The twist of fate that came about by my raising my hand that day has brought me down another path in life and a new journey. It is funny how sometimes a door opens up and when we take a reluctant step through we find something unexpectedly wonderful. This has been one of the more exciting things I have done with my career and life. I have been challenged and stimulated as never before and have pushed myself as never before. Over the next year I completed the Vodder certification process through the Vodder School of North America, attended other breast cancer conferences, read everything I could get my hands on, gave in-services to different groups who needed to have this information, and developed two different programs— one in the large HMO that trained and supported me in this program and a second in the small private-practice physical therapy clinic my husband owns. I was finally feeling like I could back off and take a deep breath when I was approached about getting involved in this book.

I am thrilled to work with patients with lymphedema. I have never worked in therapy with tools and techniques so effective (they work for almost everyone) and so needed by a group of patients who previously have had little that they could do, nor have I ever worked with a group of patients so motivated to do something to help themselves. After working with patients with primarily chronic pain for twenty years, I realized that patients who have had cancer are very special people indeed and often have a very different view of life than those with chronic pain. Many have truly been transformed by their experiences and view the world differently. It has been a gift to meet and work with so many of them.

I have only scratched the surface in the lymphedema arena. New information and research are coming out every day. I realize there is even more to learn and understand. I agreed to become involved in the writing of this book because I saw the huge need there was for people to know that there is more they can do and that help is indeed available.

In reading this, my hope is that you will find something that will help you. You need to pick out the parts that apply to you, try different things, and see what works. My belief is that each person should learn as much as possible to better understand the process of lymphedema and the treatments that are available. Then do what is necessary to effectively manage the lymphedema at a level you are comfortable with, so you can get on with your life. Much of the manual lymph drainage/lymphatic massage training I received dictates that patients do A-B-C in that order and only in that order to get the best results possible, and that anything less cannot bring good results. I have come to realize that this is not an exact science and there needs to be some flexibility to the program. No two patients, or their needs and goals, are exactly the same. Make your management of lymphedema fit you and your situation.

About the Consultants for This Book

Stephen Chandler, M.D. Dr. Chandler attended the University of McGill Medical School in Montreal and completed an internship while on rotation at the University of California County Hospital. He spent three years during the Vietnam War as a flight surgeon on air evacuations. He completed a residency in internal medicine at the University of Oregon Health Sciences University, where he also had a fellowship in hematology. In addition to his regular oncology practice, he administers to peoples of other countries through groups such as Physicians for Social Responsibility and Northwest Medical teams. In this role he has traveled throughout the world to Jamaica, Bolivia, Nicaragua, Russia, Botswana, and Finland.

Michael Goldman, M.D. Dr. Goldman earned his medical degree at New York Medical College, interned at Harbor General Hospital in Torrance, California, and did his residency at UCLA in Radiation Oncology. He has been practicing in Oregon since 1977.

James A. Schwarz, M.D. Dr. Schwarz attended college at Princeton, received his medical degree from the Medical School at the University of California in San Francisco, and did his surgical residency at Stanford. He continued with a Surgery Oncology fellowship at Roswell Park Cancer Center in Buffalo, New York. Since 1988, he has had a General Surgery practice in San Jose, California, and in Oregon. The largest portion of his practice serves oncology patients.

Part One

◆

Lymphedema:
What It Is and
How to Prevent It

1

Lymphedema

OUR LYMPHATIC SYSTEMS are vast and extremely complex. In this chapter we will discuss what comprises the lymphatic system and the causes of lymphedema in terms that can be understood by most everyone. Even with the focus on simplicity, the discussion will be somewhat technical. Do not be discouraged if it doesn't make sense entirely. In later chapters, you will see that understanding your entire system is not essential in order to successfully deal with lymphedema. Skim this section if you like, and read it again later when you can take it all in.

What Is Lymphedema?

Lymphedema is swelling, usually in the arms or legs, that occurs as a result of an impaired lymphatic system.[1] A lymphatic system can be impaired in a variety of ways: by surgery, radiotherapy, injury, or even infection. Or you can come by this impairment simply from the makeup of your genes.

The lymphatics are part of your immune system. You will see in more detail in the next chapter that they are responsible for cleansing your tissues and maintaining the balance of fluids in your system.

Specifically, the lymphatic vessels drain fluid from the tissue cells in the body, along with protein molecules, bacteria, cellular waste products, and other unusable matter. This protein-rich fluid, called *lymph* once it is in the lymphatic system, travels in one direction: toward the heart. It is transported through the lymphatic vessels to the lymph nodes, where it is filtered and cleansed before returning to the venous system and moving on to the heart. In the heart, the fluid is simply returned to the blood to be recirculated in the body.

If the lymphatic system has been impaired, the protein-rich fluid can become backed up. Swelling occurs when the amount of fluid in an area is greater than the capacity of the lymphatic system to transport it away.[2] Lymphedema has also been defined as "an abnormal accumulation of tissue proteins, edema, and chronic inflammation within an extremity."[3]

If untreated, this backed-up protein-rich fluid can provide a culture medium for bacteria that can result in infection[1] and can delay wound healing, because less oxygen gets to the tissue cells. A long-term accumulation of this fluid eventually results in thick and hardened tissues (fibrosis), which creates further resistance to draining the fluid from the limb.

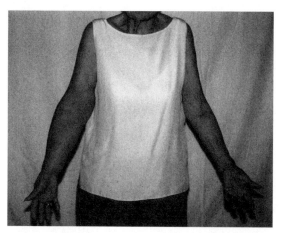

Figure 1-1. Patient with lymphedema of the right arm

If your lymph nodes are removed or radiated as part of your cancer treatment, you will be at risk for developing lymphedema for the rest of your life. In some people, the swelling starts immediately following surgery or radiotherapy. For others, it may not appear until many years later.[4] Still others may have an occurrence for a few weeks that then goes away and may or may not ever return. Sometimes extensive trauma can be the contributing factor. At other times it might be a small, inconsequential injury, such as a cat scratch or bug bite.

A woman who came into Gwen's clinic had had bilateral mastectomies, the first in 1957, the second in 1964. She had experienced no swelling problems for thirty-three years—in fact, she had no idea she even had a chance of developing lymphedema. Then, during a hot summer day when she was fixing up her home and yard to prepare for a move, packing and moving boxes, she suddenly developed lymphedema. Perhaps if she had spaced these activities out over several days, done only one of them, or done them during the coolest part of the day, she might have never developed it at all.

Types of Lymphedema

Lymphedema can occur in anyone—men, women, or children—and can have different causes. It can occur anywhere in the body, but it is most common in the arms and legs, as well as in breast tissue.

Some of the causes of lymphedema are:[5]

- Surgery, particularly when lymph nodes are removed after treatment of cancer: breast, prostate, gynecological, head or neck, colon, or melanoma.

- Radiotherapy—this kills tumor cells, but it can also cause scar tissue that interrupts the normal flow of the lymphatic system.

- Trauma that disrupts an area of lymph nodes.

- Infections, lymphangitis.

- Filariasis, a disease found mostly in endemic areas of Southeast Asia, India, and Africa, caused by parasitic worms called filaria entering the peripheral lymphatic vessels.

- Paralysis or immobility.

- Chronic venous insufficiency.

When lymphedema occurs from any of these causes it is known as *secondary lymphedema*.

Not everyone who undergoes surgical removal of lymph nodes or radiotherapy develops lymphedema. In many people the remaining lymphatics dilate or form collateral circulation or new pathways.[6] Dr. James Schwarz, a surgeon Gwen works with, says that the lymphatic system is highly variable from person to person: "This may help to explain why, of many women who have the same surgery and treatment, some develop trouble with lymphedema and some don't."[7]

There is another type of lymphedema, not associated with surgery or radiotherapy, that can be caused by a malformation or malfunction of the lymphatic system. This is known as *primary lymphedema*. It can be present at birth (Milroy's disease), develop at or around the age of puberty (lymphedema praecox), or develop after the age of thirty-five (lymphedema tarda). It is most commonly related to having too few lymphatic vessels; however, it is unclear whether people are born with this insufficiency or if it develops over time. Some suggest that the defect may be programmed at birth to cause atrophy or early aging in the lymphatic vessels, resulting in inadequate drainage.[4] In Milroy's disease, which is an inherited disorder, there is a complete absence of the initial lymph vessels.[8]

Primary lymphedema affects females more than males. In 95 percent of cases, swelling occurs in the legs, but it can develop anywhere in the body where structural abnormalities may be compromising lymph drainage. Primary lymphedema may be linked to heredity, or to genetic syndromes, and it can also develop without any genetic component.

Almost all the treatment and recommendations suggested in this book can be applied to both primary and secondary lymphedema. However, we will be concentrating on secondary lymphedema, particularly when it is found in the upper body and occurs after treatment for breast cancer.

Breast Cancer Surgery and the Lymph Nodes

Since the early 1900s, and up until recent decades, the standard treatment for breast cancer consisted of a radical mastectomy: removing the breast, muscles of the chest wall and sometimes underlying tissues, skin, and the lymph nodes in the armpit and even above the collarbone. This decreased the local recurrence of cancer and increased survival rates.

In recent decades, treatment has evolved toward more conservative surgery. In the modified radical mastectomy, the muscles of the chest wall are preserved. In breast conservation surgeries (lumpectomies), cancerous lumps are removed and fewer lymph nodes are taken out than in the radical mastectomy.[9]

Axillary Node Dissection

Axillary node dissection, or removal of lymph nodes in the armpit, is performed in most types of breast cancer surgeries to determine the extent and progression of breast cancer. It helps the medical team decide which types of postsurgical treatment to recommend. The status of the axillary lymph nodes is the single most important predictor of survival from breast cancer.[10]

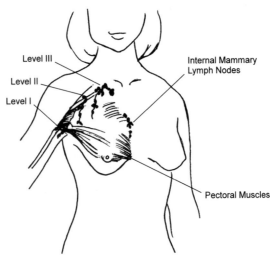

Figure 1-2. Levels of Lymph Node Dissection

Three types of axillary node dissection can be done:

1. Level I: Lymph nodes at the side edge of the breast in the armpit are removed.

2. Level II: Lymph nodes of Level I plus those behind the pectoralis minor muscle are removed.

3. Level III: Lymph nodes around the clavicle are removed.

It is most common now to remove only the nodes at Level I and II. Dr. Schwarz explains why: "Removal of nodes at level III increases the risk of further destruction of lymphatics and increases the risk of lymphedema. It is rarely done except in cases where level I and II are highly involved in the cancer. The level I and II dissection will remove most, if not all, the lymph nodes that may be involved in cancer."

Many doctors thought that there was no therapeutic value to removing lymph nodes and did it mostly to determine the extent of the cancer in order to plan treatment. Some women with lymphedema bemoan the fact that doctors removed their lymph nodes only to find that there was no cancer in the nodes. However, more recent evidence shows that even when lymph nodes test negative, a preventive dissection does indeed increase survival rates.[9]

There are some situations in which axillary node dissection may not be needed, such as with a small carcinoma in situ (cancer that has not spread to neighboring tissues). In this case, the risk of lymph node involvement is less than 1 percent, and it may be possible to avoid lymph node dissection. Dr. Schwarz suggests that there may be other cases in which axillary node dissection is not done as well, such as for an elderly woman with a slow-growing tumor or a when a woman chooses to have radiotherapy without axillary node dissection.

Clinical Examination

Surgeons have explored other ways to determine lymph node involvement that may not be as invasive or as apt to lead to ongoing problems. They can perform a physical exam in which they palpate the underarm area in patients with breast cancer. But, as Dr. Schwarz explains, even when there is cancer in the lymph nodes, the doctor cannot feel any abnormal nodes in the axilla 30 to 35 percent of the time.[7] So the method cannot be used to accurately determine axillary lymph node involvement.

Sentinel Node Biopsy

Sentinel node biopsy is a major advance in alternatives to axillary node dissection. In this procedure, a dye is injected into the breast around the tumor. The dye is followed to the first node that picks it up. This first node, the sentinel node, is then surgically removed and examined. If there is no evidence of malignancy, no more nodes are removed and axillary node dissection can be avoided. If the node is positive, the axillary node dissection can then be performed. This procedure, which can be used as a diagnostic tool, has the potential to decrease the number of axillary node dissections. However, while sentinel node biopsy has great potential, it is not yet standard practice. Dr. Schwarz outlines some reasons for this, citing a study by Armando Giuliano:

◆ The results vary greatly depending on the surgeon performing the procedure.

◆ The procedure still has too high a degree of false negatives (the sentinel node biopsied may show no cancer even when there is cancer in other nodes) for it to be standard protocol.[11]

There are also some situations in which sentinel node biopsy is not recommended:[9]

◆ When the breast cancer has been biopsied, in which case it is not as amenable to accurate sentinel node biopsy.

◆ When there is a large tumor or there are multiple sites of cancer.

◆ When there is clinical evidence of axillary node involvement.

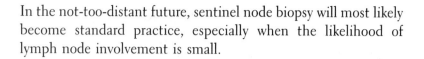

In the not-too-distant future, sentinel node biopsy will most likely become standard practice, especially when the likelihood of lymph node involvement is small.

Radiotherapy

Radiotherapy is an essential part of the treatment program for most patients who develop invasive breast cancer.[12] However, radiotherapy may increase the chance of developing lymphedema. Dr. Michael Goldman, a practicing radiation oncologist, says: "Radiotherapy doesn't prevent cancer, but it treats whatever cancer may remain after surgery and chemotherapy. The chest wall, as well as lymph nodes, may have residual cancer even after surgery and chemotherapy."[13]

He explains that radiotherapy protocols vary with each patient. Several factors are weighed in the decision of whether or not to irradiate. Radiotherapy most likely will be recommended to patients at high risk for recurrence of cancer, such as those who have large or aggressive tumors. It is also recommended for those whose lymph nodes have cancer cells in them or who show an incidence of microscopic residual disease after surgery. Dr. Goldman adds, "In most cases when a lumpectomy is performed, radiotherapy is given to the rest of the breast tissue. Without radiotherapy there is greater risk for cancer to recur. Even after modified radical mastectomy, radiation is recommended if the patient is at high risk."

It has been well documented that the development of lymphedema after breast cancer surgery and radiotherapy is related to the extent of the lymph node dissection, the extent of the breast surgery, and whether radiotherapy is given to the axilla. The more conservative the treatment, the less incidence there is of lymphedema. When breast conservation surgery is done without radiotherapy or axillary node dissection, there is no incidence of lymphedema. Adding axillary node dissection increases the incidence to 2 to 27 percent, and adding axillary radiotherapy increases it even further, to 9 to 36 percent.[12]

How Radiotherapy Affects the Lymphatic System

Lymph nodes are radiosensitive. Radiotherapy depletes the lymphocytes in the nodes and decreases their filtering function and immune function. Dr. Goldman adds that after radiotherapy, "we know the nodes don't work as well in terms of immune function," though he stresses that this affects only the arm where the nodes have been irradiated, and not the overall immune system. "The nodes are scarred by radiation and become what we call fibrotic. When they are scarred, the potential for blockage increases." That scarring process can continue for up to a year after the treatment and can be the final insult to a system that is already compromised, allowing the lymphedema to develop.

It is interesting that the lymphatic vessels themselves are resistant to radiotherapy, and their structure and function appear to remain intact even when radiated.[12] The problem arises as the surrounding tissue develops fibrosis, which interrupts the drainage of lymph vessels and can lead to lymphedema.

Choosing Breast Cancer Treatments

Given the risk of lymphedema, people with breast cancer may question whether it is advisable to pursue the more aggressive treatment. But, while cancer kills, lymphedema very rarely does. With proper attention some lymphedema can be prevented, and what can't be prevented can be effectively managed with appropriate treatment. It cannot be emphasized too strongly that the *benefits of radiotherapy far outweigh the potential risks of lymphedema*. Research clearly shows that radiotherapy improves survival rates. It also shows that radiotherapy enhances the survival benefit of chemotherapy after breast cancer surgery.[12]

Dr. Schwarz reports, "In our facility right now, women with lymph nodes testing positive for breast cancer are getting dissection *plus* radiation." He cites an article in the July 1998 *Oncology*[14] that says that radiating the lymph nodes benefits your entire system, reducing recurrences by as much as 20 to 30 percent, no matter how many nodes were involved with cancer.[14]

Dr. Schwarz concludes that there may be fewer lymph node dissections performed in the future, but that there is the possibility that more radiotherapy will be used for treatment as we learn more about what most effectively influences survival rates. Perhaps we will even become more skilled at identifying who requires what level of treatment, so axillary lymph node treatment can be minimized.

For the near future, at any rate, treatment for breast cancer will continue to incorporate methods that put us at risk for developing lymphedema. We all need to understand that, until recently, there has been too little known about lymphedema and too little attention paid to it. Dr. Goldman acknowledged this lack of knowledge when he said, "Some patients think lymphedema is caused by their bodies making too much fluid."

No matter how overwhelmed we may be by the diagnosis of cancer, no matter how dismayed at the choices we are required to consider, we must take lymphedema into account—not in order to refuse treatment, but because the more educated our decisions, the less chance we may have of future complications. Information is the key. In chapter 6 we will discuss what you can do to prevent lymphedema, and in part 2 we will discuss the many things you can do to treat it.

2

The Lymphatic System

ALTHOUGH YOUR LYMPHATIC SYSTEM is vast and complex, your ability to treat lymphedema does not depend on understanding it. If you want, skip this technical section and get right to learning how to treat your lymphedema. As with chapter 1, you can always come back and read this later.

In order to understand lymphedema it is helpful to first understand the normal lymphatic system. The lymphatic system is a part of the circulatory system, but unlike the blood system it works according to a "one-way" principle: it carries its load of fluid and waste products in only one direction, from the tissue cells in the body to the heart, filtering and cleansing the load in the lymph nodes along the way.[1] The waste products are broken down in the lymph nodes to a form that can be safely excreted from the body. Once it reaches the heart, the lymph fluid joins the blood to increase blood volume. The next illustration shows the extensive lymphatic system with its complex network of superficial and deep vessels and lymph nodes.

The lymphatic system has several important functions:

♦ It maintains fluid balance in the body by collecting excess fluid that is not absorbed by the blood capillaries and transporting it back to the heart.

♦ It removes proteins, impurities, waste products, and bacteria from the tissues throughout the body.

♦ It filters the impurities and concentrates the fluid as it passes through the lymph nodes.

◆ It participates in creating antibodies (cells called B-cells and T-cells, or lymphocytes and thymocytes) that are custom-designed to fight infection and foreign protein.

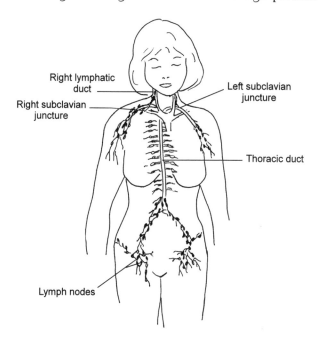

Figure 2-1. Lymphatic Pathways and Regional Lymph Nodes

Lymphatic Vessels

The lymphatic vessels begin as fingerlike capillaries between cells in the interstitial tissue (the space between tissues).[2] It may help to think of the tissue cells as marbles in a jar. The interstitial space is the space between the marbles; the interstitial fluid fills that space.

The blood arterial capillaries (small arteries that carry blood from the heart) bring fluid and nutrients into the interstitial spaces and to the tissue cells. Ninety percent of the fluid is reabsorbed by the venous capillaries (small veins that carry blood back to the heart). The lymphatic capillaries absorb the 10 percent excess fluid left behind in the interstitial space, along with protein molecules, bacteria and viruses, and other waste products.[3]

Returning to our analogy of marbles in a jar, most of this fluid between the marbles is removed by the blood capillaries, but some of the fluid remains, along with protein molecules and waste materials that are too large for the blood capillaries to absorb. This is what the lymphatic capillaries absorb.

How Does the Fluid Get into the Lymphatic Capillaries?

The lymph capillaries have a slightly larger diameter than blood capillaries and have a unique structure that permits fluid to flow into them. When the pressure is greater in the interstitial fluid than in the initial lymph vessel, the cell flaps of the initial lymph vessel separate slightly (like the opening of a one-way valve), and fluid enters the lymphatic capillary. As the vessel fills, the tissue pressure decreases and the valve closes.[2] Once the interstitial fluid enters the lymphatic capillary, it is called *lymph*.[1]

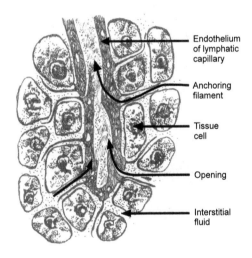

Endothelium
of lymphatic
capillary

Anchoring
filament

Tissue
cell

Opening

Interstitial
fluid

Figure 2-2. Initial Lymph Vessel

The lymph capillaries collect fluid from small interstitial areas and gradually join together into bigger lymph vessels called collecting vessels. Most of the lymphatic vessels have valves that prevent backflow of fluid. A single segment along the collector from valve to valve is called the *lymph angion*.

The vessels become progressively larger as they converge and approach the lymph nodes. After being filtered through the lymph nodes, the lymph eventually drains into the larger lymphatic trunks and ultimately into the veins at the lower neck.[1] Over two-thirds of the lymph from the body drains into the large thoracic duct (the main lymphatic vessel in your trunk) and into the left subclavian (under the collarbone) vein at your neck.

How Does the Lymph Fluid Move?

Once fluid picked up from the body's tissue enters the lymphatic vessels, it is moved through the vessel/node system by several driving forces. Within the lymphatic system itself the fluid, now called lymph, is transported by:[3]

1. The random contraction of the smooth muscle wall of the lymph vessel: these contractions push fluid through the vessels six to seven times a minute. The valves located inside the collectors allow lymph flow in only one direction.

2. A stretch reflex of the angions: when one angion fills, it causes a stretch to the next angion, which will then contract and move the fluid through the next angion.

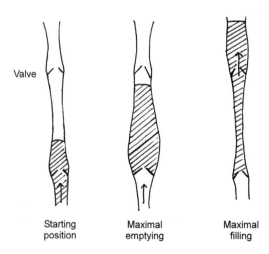

Valve

Starting position

Maximal emptying

Maximal filling

Figure 2-3. Lymph Angions

Besides the lymph system, other actions influence the lymph vessels:

- The pumping of the arterial system.

- The pumping of the muscles.

- Abdominal breathing, which causes a change in pressure of the chest cavity, stimulating the central thoracic duct.

- Peristalsis, or the rolling action of the intestines.

- Manual lymphatic massage.

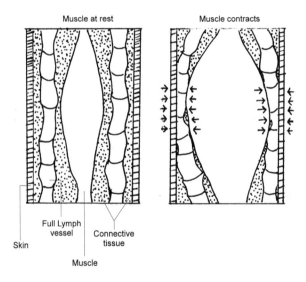

Fig 2-4. Muscle Pump

Because all these actions affect the lymph vessels, these are also areas where you can take action to improve the efficiency of your lymph vessels and treat your lymphedema. We will look at these options in part 2, under treatments.

Lymph Nodes

Lymph nodes are kidney-bean-shaped structures located along

the lymphatic vessels. Between five hundred and fifteen hundred of them are scattered throughout the body, but they are most heavily concentrated in areas such as the axilla (in the armpit), groin, mammary glands, and neck.

The lymph nodes have two main functions. First, they produce lymphocytes, which are white blood cells that combat infection by producing antibodies to fight bacteria and viruses. Second, they filter lymph, destroying and removing dead cells, waste materials, protein molecules, bacteria, and viruses. When the lymph nodes are functioning correctly, lymphatic fluid is cleaned and fortified, ready to be returned to the blood.

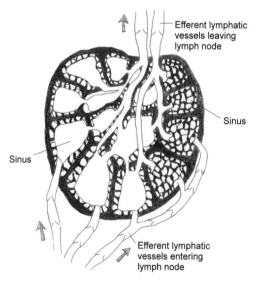

Figure 2-5. Lymph Node Structure

Dr. Michael Goldman says, "The lymph node acts as a trap, trapping infection." He goes on to say, "When the lymph node has infection, antibodies are triggered to counteract that protein. Then, when infection disappears, most of those particular cells disappear as well. But a few remain in case there is another need later on."

The lymph nodes house the T-lymphocytes and B-lymphocytes, which are important in supporting the immune system because they produce customized agents to counteract infection and other foreign material.[4]

The lymph nodes do not regenerate when they are removed or if they are damaged by radiotherapy. In other words, the lymph nodes cannot repair themselves. However, researchers have identified a growth factor, VEGF-C, that appears to induce the enlargement of lymphatic vessels. This has potential for improving healing after breast cancer treatment if the lymphatic vessels remaining are able to carry larger volumes of fluid.[5]

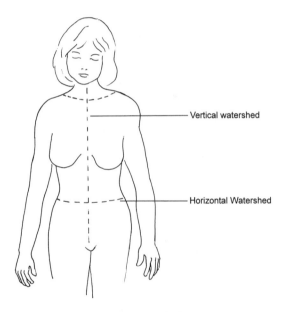

Vertical watershed

Horizontal Watershed

Figure 2-6. Watersheds

Watersheds

The watersheds are the boundaries between the areas of lymph drainage. The body is divided by three watersheds, a vertical one and a horizontal one, which results in four quarters (see Figure 2.6 above), as well as another one for the head and neck. We will refer to each quarter as a *quadrant*. These quadrants are particularly important in the drainage techniques used to move fluid in lymphedema treatment, which redirects fluid from an ineffective quadrant to a healthy adjacent quadrant where the fluid can be normally drained and filtered.[6] We will discuss them in more detail in the chapters on treating lymphedema.

These watershed boundaries are similar to watersheds on the tops of mountains (one patient referred to her vertical watershed as the Continental Divide), in that water flows one way if you are on one side of the mountain's watershed and flows the other way once you cross the divide. There are small lymphatic vessels that cross the watershed and can transport lymph from one quadrant to another.

3

Signs of Lymphedema

SEVERAL SIGNS CAN INDICATE that you might have the initial onset
of lymphedema. If you notice any of the signs given below, or
even if you are concerned that you might develop lymphedema,
call your doctor or contact the National Lymphedema Network
(see chapter 28, "Where to Get Help"). Though women who
have had lymphedema for many years have achieved relief after
treatment, the sooner lymphedema is treated, the better the
chance of reducing the swelling.[1]

Some signs to look for are:[2]

- A feeling of fullness or pressure, which can be the first sign
  of swelling.

- The sensation of swelling, which can often be present even
  before swelling can be seen. Edema is not detectable clin-
  ically until interstitial volume reaches 30 percent above
  normal.[3] Also, 50 percent of people with visible arm lymphedema report that the first symptom was a feeling of
  heaviness and fullness in the arm.[4]

- Puffiness, swelling, or any increase in the size of the limb
  or anywhere in the quarter of your body that has had surgery or radiotherapy. That swelling can be in your armpit
  (axilla), on part of your chest, or around the scar areas, as
  well as the arm.

- A pins-and-needles sensation in the limb.

- A feeling of heat in your arm or in the affected side of
  your body.

❖ Redness and inflammation (this may indicate infection, so see your doctor right away).

❖ Pitting: if you press the skin and hold it in a moment, the skin does not bounce back.

❖ A "bursting" sensation in the limb.

❖ Aching in the limb, in the shoulder, or in back of your shoulder.

❖ The inability to pinch a fold of skin of one of your fingers between your finger and thumb.

The International Society of Lymphology has graded lymphedema into categories:[5]

In Grade 1, when the skin is pressed (as mentioned above), the pressure will leave a pit that takes some time to fill back in. This is referred to as *pitting edema*. Sometimes the swelling can be reduced by elevating the limb for a few hours. There is little or no fibrosis (hardening) at this stage, so it is usually reversible.

In Grade 2 lymphedema, when the swollen area is pressed, it does not pit, and the swelling is not reduced very much by elevation. If left untreated, the tissue in the limb gradually hardens and becomes fibrotic.

In Grade 3, the lymphedema is often called *elephantiasis*. It occurs almost exclusively in the legs after progressive, long-term, and untreated lymphedema. At this stage there may be gross changes to the skin and it may protrude and bulge. There may be some leakage of fluid through the tissue in the affected area, especially if there is a cut or sore. While lymphedema will respond to treatment at this stage, it is rarely reversible.

Diagnosing Lymphedema

There is no way to predict if, when, or where in the quadrant of your body affected by surgery and radiation, you may develop lymphedema. It is not unusual for lymphedema to begin long after you have finished having regular and frequent appointments with your doctor. Dr. Stephen Chandler, in his medical oncology practice, tells of one patient who didn't have lymphedema for many years after dissection. "She came to me after one powerful winter storm when she developed swelling after lifting bales of hay for her farm animals." He encourages patients to pay attention to changes in their bodies and adds that it is often up to the patient to notice when help may be needed.

Usually, a diagnosis of lymphedema can be easily made by your doctor taking a complete history and conducting a thorough physical examination. But there are some diagnostic tests, such as lymphoscintigraphy, MRI, and CT scans (which can accurately visualize the lymphatics), which can aid in the diagnosis. It may be helpful to seek a referral to a specialist in lymphology if, after a physical exam, the diagnosis is still unclear or in need of further documentation.[6] One test that used to be done involved injecting a contrast medium into the lymphatics, then taking X-rays (lymphangiography). This test has been discontinued, in most cases, as it can cause damage to the remaining lymphatics.

Though there are many things you can do to try to prevent the onset of lymphedema (see chapter 7, "Preventing Lymphedema"), if you have had surgery and radiotherapy to the lymph nodes you are considered vulnerable. It is important to know and watch for the symptoms and, if you suspect you are experiencing some of them, contact your doctor right away. If you do have lymphedema, the sooner you begin treatment, the better.

4

Incidence of Lymphedema After Breast Cancer

STUDIES OF HOW MANY PEOPLE develop lymphedema after breast cancer show great variation, with reported incidence ranging from 7 to 70 percent.[1] Dr. Susan Love, in the 1995 edition of Dr. Susan Love's Breast Book, says she believes lymphedema occurs in only about 10 percent of mastectomies, but she goes on to say, "I think, however, that this figure is a bit low, and that if we measured every patient carefully in the follow-up visits we'd find the mild cases are a lot more common."[2] A recent study cited in the New England Journal of Medicine says the figure is 60 percent for women who have had radical mastectomies and 30 percent for those who have had modified mastectomies or breast-conserving surgeries.[3]

Dr. Stephen Chandler indicates that he sees a wide range in the incidence of lymphedema in his medical oncology practice. "I think it's possible that right after dissection every woman develops some degree of lymphedema," he says. "With some, the edema is apparent, but with others it isn't. The lymphatics are so small and fragile. I see many patients for lymphedema after surgery, not to mention those I see after radiation therapy. I think radiation may lead to as much, or more, edema than is caused by surgery." While lymphedema can happen at any time after treatment for cancer, Dr. Chandler commonly sees women developing lymphedema four to six months after treatment.

Dr. Judith Casley-Smith, world-recognized authority in the field of lymphedema, suggests one-third of all patients develop lymphedema after mastectomy.[4] In a recent review of 272 women treated for breast cancer in the late 1970s, clinicians from Memorial Sloan Kettering Cancer Center in New York found that most of the women reported some symptoms of lymphedema.[5] A more recent review of seven studies from around the world showed that the incidence of lymphedema ranges from 6 to 30 percent. Another study showed that 28 percent of patients had measurable lymphedema after breast cancer treatment—*measurable*, in that study, being defined as the affected arm being greater in circumference than the contralateral arm by two inches or more. However, in that same study, an additional 17 percent said their arms "felt" swollen even if there was no measurable difference.[6]

Almost all studies in the past ten years correlate the incidence and degree of lymphedema to the general extent of the surgical dissection.[7] But axillary radiation therapy also increases the incidence of lymphedema.

Dr. Michael Goldman says, "The greater the amount of lymph nodes removed, the greater the risk for lymphedema. Patients who have simple lumpectomies and radiotherapy only to the chest wall, without lymph node radiotherapy or dissection, rarely develop lymphedema." Dr. Goldman adds that he may not follow people for a long time after their treatment with radiation, so it is difficult for him to predict when someone might develop lymphedema.[8]

It is important to note that men can also develop breast cancer and have similar treatment with surgery, radiotherapy, and chemotherapy. While it is much less common for men than women, and statistically very rare, most people are not aware that breast cancer can occur in men. Often their cancer is not detected until it has progressed to a later stage of the disease, which requires more extensive treatment. Men with lymph node dissection or radiotherapy have the same risk as women for developing lymphedema. Gwen has seen several men in her clinic after breast cancer treatment; two of them developed lymphedema after strenuous activity. They had never heard of lymphedema before and were not aware of any precautions to follow. Their treatment was the same as for women who develop lymphedema.

Why the Wide Range in Statistics?

Reports of the incidence of lymphedema after breast cancer vary so widely because there are no clear standards or uniform diagnostic criteria for measuring it.[6] Some doctors define lymphedema as two centimeters greater circumference of the involved arm, others say three centimeters, still others say two inches.

Other factors include the prolonged time periods involved, since lymphedema may develop many years after the treatment of cancer; lack of contact with the original surgeon or oncologist; the view of some medical providers that lymphedema is less important than eradicating cancer and detecting recurrence;[9] and, finally, underreporting of lymphedema and its symptoms by patients. Many women may not report the symptoms of lymphedema, especially if they think there is nothing that can be done for it. In a mailed questionnaire to women after breast cancer, a survey found that half of the patients who reported swelling did not report it to their doctor.[6]

Doctors Downplay Lymphedema

In the past, doctors generally have not been very supportive of patients with lymphedema and have minimized the problems it poses. Carolyn Renowicz, M.D., director of the Division of Gynecological Oncology at Albert Einstein College of Medicine, says, "Some doctors trivialize lymphedema, dismissing it as 'just a little swelling' that is a small price to pay for cancer treatment."[1]

Many doctors believe the swelling isn't lymphedema unless the arm is *really* big, and only then might they mention to patients that something should be done. Often physicians do not even recognize the lymphedema that appears in the trunk or breast. Others suggest their patients learn to live with the condition, as there is nothing to be done about it.[10]

There is a serious lack of medical expertise in the diagnosis and treatment of lymphedema. Many surgeons believe very few patients actually develop lymphedema; however, it is more likely that by the time many women develop lymphedema, their condition is no longer being monitored by their surgeon. Dr. Chandler agrees, indicating that he feels the medical community has downplayed lymphedema. "Until recently," he says, "there just wasn't anything to do for it."

The view that lymphedema is not important is changing as doctors begin to recognize the medical as well as psychosocial and emotional complications of untreated lymphedema. But such change is very recent. Even in the 1995 edition of Dr. Susan Love's *Breast Book*, only 3 out of 611 pages mention lymphedema; and Dr. Love states that there is not much you can do about it.[2] In the past, patients with lymphedema had few treatment options, but now, new treatment methodologies have been developed.

Lymphedema Is Serious

Lymphedema *is* a very serious condition. It frequently results in complications, such as lymphangitis (a bacterial infection of the lymphatic system), skin changes, fibrosis, and infection. There are less common, life-threatening complications as well, such as the development of a rare type of cancer, lymphangiosarcoma, in the affected arm. This can occur in patients with long-term, untreated, or improperly treated lymphedema (after eight to ten years).[11] Unfortunately, this condition requires immediate amputation.

Lymphedema may worsen with time if it is left untreated. It can become disabling by stiffening joints or making the limbs heavy and cumbersome, and may cause significant cosmetic deformities. Lymphedema can also have huge psychological, social, and emotional effects on the woman who develops it. If the swelling is great enough, it can't be hidden. In fact, a swollen arm is far more visible than the loss of a breast.[6]

The debate about the percentage of women who develop lymphedema continues, but no matter what the statistics say, if you have lymphedema, you want help. In spite of what doctors have historically maintained, there is something you can do about it, and we will get into that in great detail soon.

But first, here is the first of our personal stories of living with lymphedema. We'll meet Jean, a physical therapist assistant whose lymphedema began, in typical fashion, long after her cancer treatment. Jean's story shows how it is possible to live a full and active life by taking care of yourself and treating your lymphedema.

5

Jean: A Physical Therapist Assistant Deals with Her Own Lymphedema

JEAN IS SIXTY-ONE. She is a short woman, round-faced and square of build. She is wearing a handmade sweater with a rose design along the shoulder. Her complexion is smooth and her smile brisk and ready.

Jean works four days a week as a physical therapist assistant at the same health facility where her breast cancer was diagnosed and where she had a lumpectomy four years ago. In the last six months she has been working part-time, assisting with patients who have lymphedema. "I was going to retire," she says, "but the choice to work with lymphedema patients was too interesting, so I didn't. I'll wait to retire."

Jean's own problems with lymphedema started about a year and a half earlier, two years after her chemotherapy and radio-therapy. She said she did some heavy housework one day and then took a very hot bath. She emerged from the tub with a swollen arm. By then, she was living alone, because halfway through her chemotherapy, her husband left her. "Everything happened at once," she says, "moving from the house we'd lived in for twenty years, the cancer, and my husband leaving." Then she chuckles, "You can get a lot accomplished with personal growth when that happens."

"Halfway through chemo, after my husband left, I just sort of fell apart." Like everything else this is said without rancor, but with a sort of ironic humor.

Her sweater is pulled halfway up her forearm, the arm with the lymphedema. It is noticeably larger than the other. As if she has just noticed her arm, she says, "I've been helping my daughter move." She presses her fingers into the underside of her forearm. When she removes them, there are four deep crescents. "I guess I need to bandage for a couple of days," she says. (Compression treatments like bandaging are discussed later, in chapters 14–18.) "I do that when my arm puffs like this.

"Anyway," she says, "when everything happened, I had every opportunity to fix what was broken. I worked in health care. And did I put the system to use!" She laughs. "I went to all kinds of counselors. I thought that maybe since I'd always been the type to hold everything in, maybe it could have caused my cancer, and I wanted to learn not to hold *anything* in anymore. I just didn't have time to die. I wanted to see my grandchild. I just had too much to do.

"I always wanted to square dance, so I took lessons, even though I didn't have a husband to do it with. And I had a wonderful time.

"Well," she says, "You'll never guess what happened. My husband and I started dating. By then I had stuff pretty much together, I mean, about the cancer and the loneliness without him. He was living across town but spending most of his time with me. I knew I wanted someone in my life and I began to realize I didn't want to go on forever like we were, so one night I told him, 'Either you come home or I want a divorce, and I don't think I'm going to want to see you again.' I wasn't mad. I wasn't trying to hold on to him or to anyone. I just wanted to get on with my life." She grins and gives a flip to her eyebrows. "He came home."

Her mood grows serious for a moment. "I have something to say, something that really bugs me: I *hate* to be called a cancer survivor because that implies I am a victim of cancer. I'm not a victim. I just had cancer, that's all. I want to get on with my life. I want to *do* something about it, not *think* about it. To me, working with lymphedema treatment is doing something. See, I'm only sixty-one. I still have some life. I'd love to be part of a lymphedema treatment clinic for low-income women who can't afford treatments. I could show them how to bandage and how to take care of themselves, maybe even teach them to team up and to massage each other for treatment. It's something I want to do when I'm retired.

"You know," she says, referring to some of the most common self-help treatments, "I've noticed that our patients who do the exercises, who do the self-massages, who get out and live life, who walk, swim, ride bikes—they are the ones who manage okay with lymphedema. It's the ones who are depressed, who don't finish their series of treatments, who sort of give up, they're the ones who really end up with trouble.

"We had one woman who was eighty years old when she came in for treatment. She'd had lymphedema for several years. She was so skeptical. She couldn't believe it would work, but she kept at it and her arm came down and she quit hurting and a while back she wrote us a note. She's vacationing with her family in Kansas. Now that's what treatment can do if you let it."

6

History of Lymphedema Treatment

UNTIL RECENTLY, there were limited options available in the United States for people who developed lymphedema. Most women were told that nothing could be done for it and to just "live with it," or they were placed on a compression pump and then given a special garment to wear.

This situation is surprising, because treatment of the lymphatic system has been widely used in Europe for sixty years. Manual lymph drainage (MLD®, a light massage technique that moves lymph from one part of the body to another) was first developed in the 1930s by the late Dr. Emil Vodder and Estrid Vodder of Denmark.[1] The Vodders pioneered this work for many years, starting their work in Cannes, then moving to Paris, where the first publication about MLD® appeared in 1936. They returned to Denmark at the start of the war and founded the MLD® Institute in Copenhagen.

By 1967 a society for the Vodders' MLD® work had formed.[2] Work done in their clinic in Germany and in Europe by Drs. Ethel and Michael Foeldi in the 1970s and 1980s helped to validate the effectiveness of lymphatic massage in reducing lymphedema.[3]

During that same time, Drs. John and Judith Casley-Smith began their work with lymphedema in Australia. They have done much to enhance the field of lymphedema treatment through research, training, education, and treatment programs. In 1982, they founded the Lymphoedema Association of Australia.[4] Throughout the decades, their many publications have been well received worldwide. With the passing of Dr. John Casley-Smith, Dr. Judith Casley-Smith continues the work they began together. Guenther and Hildegarde Wittlinger, longtime pupils of Dr. Emil Vodder, founded the Dr. Vodder Schule in Austria in 1971. A Dr. Vodder School of North America was founded in the early 1990s, and under its director, Robert Harris, continues to actively train therapists throughout Canada and the United States in the use of the Vodder techniques of manual lymph drainage.

In 1988 the National Lymphedema Network, a nonprofit organization located in San Francisco, was founded by Saskia R. J. Thiadens, R.N. The organization's goal is to provide education and guidance to lymphedema patients and health care professionals around the country. Since its formation, the National Lymphedema Network has gained international recognition.[5] Ms. Thiadens has been a leader in the treatment of lymphedema in the United States, having opened one of the country's first lymphedema treatment clinics in San Francisco.

Dr. Robert Lerner, medical director of Lerner Lymphedema Services in New Jersey, New York, and Florida, brought the complete decongestive physiotherapy approach to lymphedema care to the United States from Europe in the late 1980s. He and his trained staff have been successfully treating patients ever since. He is also actively involved in the training of therapists throughout the United States.

Even with the efforts of organizations such as the National Lymphedema Network (NLN) and the practices of other competent therapists, broad knowledge of lymphedema and the effective treatments for it have been slow in coming to the medical community in the United States. Relatively few people here have been trained to carry out these treatment approaches, though more and more therapists are being certified. You can find a resource guide to the leading schools, organizations, and specialists in chapter 28, "Where to Get Help."

After all this time, comprehensive treatment involving lymphatic massaging, bandaging, exercise, and skin care is finally becoming recognized as the best approach to care for people who develop lymphedema. The International Society of Lymphology published a Consensus Document in 1995 and updated it again in 1997. The document outlined these techniques as the most effective approach to the treatment of lymphedema.[6]

And, in an important presentation to the Society of Phlebology of America, Dr. Robert Lerner summarized his results of decongestive lymphatic therapy performed on one thousand of his patients with upper extremity lymphedema. The patients were treated between 1989 and 1995. The results showed that the therapy caused an average of 62 percent reduction in volume of fluid in the arm or leg.[7]

In February 1998, the American Cancer Society, with the involvement of Saskia Thiadens, R.N., organized a workshop in New York. The workshop consisted of leading experts on lymphedema, including Ms. Thiadens, Dr. Judith Casley-Smith, Dr. Robert Lerner, Drs. Ethel and Michael Foeldi, Dr. Kasseroller, and Dr. Leduc. The participants agreed with the Society of Lymphology's recommendation of massage, bandaging, exercise, and skin care as the most effective regimen. The group, recognizing the confusion about what to call this therapeutic protocol, decided to settle on a common name, decongestive lymphatic therapy.[8]

In this book we will discuss each of the recommended parts of this treatment in detail, and you will learn how to incorporate them into your own life.

7

What Can I Do to Prevent Lymphedema?

IT IS NOT CLEARLY UNDERSTOOD why some people develop lymphedema, no matter what precautions they take, and others never develop it no matter what they do. As mentioned in the previous chapters, whether you experience lymphedema soon after treatment for cancer, or are fortunate enough never to get it, surgery and radiotherapy compromise your system and leave you with a higher risk for developing lymphedema than if you'd never had these treatments for cancer at all. It is important to try to avoid lymphedema, and we will discuss preventive methods in this chapter. If lymphedema develops despite these precautions, the beneficial habits you practice will certainly help you to manage it better.

Education is the key. Many patients who develop lymphedema report that they were unaware of the risk or how the symptoms might present themselves, nor did they have any information about precautions that might prevent it.

There is no doubt that lymphedema education is critical after surgery. But it is essential *before* surgery as well. Patients need to learn to recognize the early signs and symptoms of lymphedema and to know their importance in order to seek early and aggressive intervention and to take precautionary measures.

It should be stressed that lifelong adherence to a careful regimen is indicated, since lymphedema may occur anytime after surgery. Breast cancer survivors who follow precautions after treatment may lower their risk of developing lymphedema. In general, it is best to avoid injury, be a fanatic about good skin care, eat well, exercise, and do things in moderation. How many times in our lives have we been told *that?* Well, now it really counts. Some specific suggestions follow.[1]

Avoid Infection and Injury

This may seem obvious: we never want infection or injury. Most of us spend our lives keeping away from them. But avoiding them now is especially important.

It is important to avoid breaking the skin in the affected quadrant, as that can lead to infection. There is always bacteria covering our skin, and a break in the skin can allow the bacteria to enter. With fewer lymph nodes there is a decreased ability to fight off bacteria, and that too can lead to increased risk for infection. Developing a safer lifestyle can make all the difference.

Start by learning to change little habits: shred cheese with your unaffected hand (do you know anybody who doesn't get a nick shredding cheese?), use a drumwheel cheese grater, or buy cheese already shredded. Wear insect repellent to avoid bug bites. Wear gloves and long sleeves when you garden and do housework. Rather than cutting your cuticles, moisturize them with lotion and gently push them back. Be sure to advise anyone giving you a manicure to do this as well. If you have blood drawn, have an IV, or are given a shot, ensure that your affected side is avoided. Avoid acupuncture to the side of your body that is involved. Avoid pet scratches, or anything that can puncture or cut the skin. Use antibiotic ointment such as Neosporin or Bacitracin if you do get cut, and watch for skin changes. At first, it may take concentration to develop safer habits. One patient, who wanted to remove warts, innocently used over-the-counter wart medication. Within days she had a dramatic increase in the swelling, and her extremity has never returned to "pre-wart-removal" size.

Watch for signs of infection: rash, itching, pain, warmth, redness, streaking of color, sudden swelling, hardness, or high fever.

An infection in your arm can move quickly and become very serious in a matter of hours. If there is any sudden change in the status of your arm or you are concerned about one of these symptoms, call your doctor, who will most likely prescribe antibiotics immediately. Generally, antibiotics in the penicillin category, such as dicloxacillin or Keflex, have proven very effective, but your physician will decide which one is most likely to work for you. Infections will bring additional lymph fluid to the area. Many women have reported that their lymphedema started with an infection.[2]

While traveling outside the country, it might be advisable to carry oral antibiotics if you have been prone to infections in the past or will be traveling in an area where limited medical care is available.[3]

Avoid Pressure on the Involved Extremity

It's important to avoid any constriction on a lymphatic system that has been compromised. Constriction can eventually cause swelling in the chest wall, shoulder, or affected arm. It is critical to avoid anything that would put any pressure on the involved areas. This means having your blood pressure taken on the unaffected arm. If, because of surgery or radiotherapy, you have a compromised lymphatic system on both sides of your body, your doctor or nurse may be able to use your leg to take your blood pressure or to give you injections, although it might be challenging to convince them to follow these precautions.

Wear jewelry and watches on the unaffected arm. Even a loose bracelet or watch could potentially cause a problem if it is bumped or catches on something and causes a cut or scratch. Resting your arm against something could cause the jewelry to press against your skin. Avoid carrying your purse over your shoulder on the affected side.

Avoid Constrictive Clothing

Be careful with wrist cuffs and tight sleeves if you already have developed lymphedema. Your favorite dress may no longer be something that you can easily wear; it may cause unnecessary constriction on your arm.

A well-fitting brassiere is critical. While many women become much more relaxed about the use of brassieres after breast cancer surgery and often choose alternative undergarments that cause no constriction, the dominant feeling in our culture is that women should wear a brassiere. The July 1997 issue of the *National Lymphedema Network Newsletter*[4] contains an excellent article with guidelines regarding the use of brassieres. It suggests that anyone who has had axillary node dissection should *never* wear a brassiere with an underwire again, since this can cause constriction or even leave deep indentations that could lead to skin breakdown and possible infection. It is important to wear a brassiere with wide, adjustable straps that are padded over the shoulders to avoid pressure to the collarbone area. If there is extra tissue, called a "dog ear," below the armpit, we suggest wearing a brassiere with a wide band to support and cover the area on the side of your chest (doctors sometimes leave extra tissue on the lateral trunk wall in case the patient decides on reconstructive surgery, but this often becomes a reservoir for lymph fluid collection). Some women find that a sports bra is very comfortable and not binding in any one area.

Some department stores selling brassieres have personnel trained to assist with brassiere selection for women who have had breast cancer. Some specialty stores carry excellent products or can help with custom-made or fitted brassieres if that is necessary. In general, recommended over-the-counter brassieres include

- Bali #3821 (wireless with padded shoulder straps).

- Playtex 18-Hour #4125 (wireless with padded shoulder straps).

- Olga #35609 (lighter-weight wireless with wide straps).

- Olga #2321 (lightweight wireless with wider, lightly padded shoulder straps).

Avoid Vigorous Activity

Don't bring on muscle fatigue. If you work out, don't "go for the burn" in your affected arm—or anywhere in your body for that matter. Watch that whatever you carry is not too heavy, particularly when carried with the arm down (as with a heavy suitcase). Avoid vigorous repetitive movements against resistance with your affected arm (rubbing, scrubbing, pushing, and pulling, as with a vacuum cleaner). I suggest that women try to find someone else to help with the heavy housework, which can involve many of these movements. If you cannot convince other household members to do some of the heavy housework, or it isn't financially possible to pay someone else to do it, follow some simple precautions. If you have short stretch bandages, it may be useful to wrap your arm before you start your housework and keep it wrapped while cleaning. You get a dual benefit from this: your house will be clean and you will have effectively worked to decrease the fluid in your arm. (Bandaging will be covered in a later chapter.)

Since we don't live in a void, and for most of us at least some housework is inevitable, here are some other ideas to reduce stress to your arm:

- Use your other arm or both arms.

- Do household chores in small amounts at a time.

- Take frequent breaks.

- Use moderation as your motto and pace yourself.

- Adjust your priorities, determine what is really important. After all, what price are you willing to pay (with increased swelling in your arm) to have a clean house? Fatigue, heat, and overdoing can all bring increased blood flow to an area, causing an increase in fluid in the tissue, which can overload an impaired lymphatic system.

Directly after surgery and treatment, *gradually* return to your previous activity level, and always monitor your arm's response to it. You may want to measure your affected arm and use the measurement as a baseline to determine how your arm is doing.

Exercise Care while Shaving

Use an electric razor to shave under the affected arm. Safety razors can nick you as easily as cheese shredders, and you may not have normal sensation under that arm to alert you that you have cut yourself. The good news is that after surgery and radiotherapy, many women experience a decrease in the growth of underarm hair.

Avoid Heat

Avoid whatever will bring heat to the area: sunbathing, sunburns (use at least SPF 15 sunscreen), and heat-producing ointments like Bengay or Absorbine Jr. Try to stay out of the sun, or cover your skin on the involved areas if you are in the sun. Even a suntan, which may look healthy, is hard on the skin because it tends to dry it out. Stay out of hot tubs and saunas. Some people still go hot-tubbing and hold their affected arm outside the water, but often the temperature is so hot it will raise the temperature of your body, including the trunk on the side that drains into the armpit. One man who had had surgery and radiotherapy ten years earlier without any incidence of lymphedema was advised to use a hot Jacuzzi after a car accident. After several weeks of using a hot tub, the swelling started.

Try to take cool, not hot, baths or showers. Avoid applying heating pads or the newer fad of microwaveable rice bags to anywhere in the affected quadrant of the body—this means if you have had a back or neck strain unrelated to the breast cancer and follow-up treatment, use ice rather than heat.

Hot weather tends to cause more swelling. You may want to find a cool place to go when the temperature and humidity are the highest (like an air-conditioned bedroom). And, when it's hot, it is important to use bandages to keep the swelling down.

Keep Your Skin in Good Condition

Try to keep your skin clean, soft, and moisturized. Wash with a mild, hypoallergenic soap that will not dry your skin. After washing, dry thoroughly. If your skin is fragile, pat your arm dry rather than rubbing it. Suggested soaps include Dove, Neutrogena, Aveeno, Basis, Tone, and Oil of Olay.

After bathing, immediately apply a moisturizing lotion, preferably one without fragrance, that has a low pH and contains alpha hydroxy, or some lasting moisturizer. Eucerin Plus, Lac Hydrin 5, and Aquafor are excellent products that may have been already recommended if you have had radiotherapy. Areas that are prone to collecting moisture, such as armpits, elbows, and under the breasts, should be kept dry by applying cornstarch or powder.

Maintain Your Ideal Weight

You may have heard a million times that you should watch your weight, but fat can be a special problem with an impaired lymph system. Fat is deposited in the interstitial tissue and can make it more difficult for the fluid to pass through tissue and into the lymph vessels. The Memorial Sloan Kettering Cancer Center reviewed 272 women who had been treated for breast cancer in the 1970s. Two factors were found to be most significant in the development of lymphedema: weight gain and incidence of injury or infection to the arm.[5] More recently, at the 1998 American Cancer Society's lymphedema workshop, Dr. Allen Meek reported that lymphedema is more common in obese patients.[6] Dr. James Schwarz agrees that obesity puts a patient at higher risk for lymphedema.

While losing weight, or maintaining it, might not necessarily reduce the swelling, gaining weight can bring on an episode of swelling. Weight gain or the inability to lose weight can be an issue if you received chemotherapy or are taking tamoxifen.

Avoid Extended Use of Diuretics

Diuretics reduce the volume of swelling, and they are often the first thing that a doctor (especially a primary care physician) might think of when you consult them about swelling, but they are not helpful with lymphedema.[7] Extended use of diuretics can actually worsen the problems associated with lymphedema. They do decrease the fluid, but at the same time don't do anything with the protein, bacteria, and waste products that remain. In fact, once the fluid is reduced, there is evidence that a much higher concentration of protein remains. The elevated concentration levels can cause the tissue to become fibrotic and thickened, leading to increased problems with fluid removal.

Exercise Regularly—But Don't Overdo It

Exercise must be incorporated into all rehabilitation programs.[8] Consult your therapist about which sports and exercises are the best for you. The lymphatic system is stimulated by the pumping action of the blood vessels, as well as the pumping action of muscles, so anything you can do to improve your circulatory system will be helpful for the lymphatic system. A good exercise goal to work toward is thirty minutes three or four times a week of an activity that will mildly increase your heart rate. General aerobic guidelines are to stay within 60 to 80 percent of your maximum heart rate. To figure your own rate, subtract your age from 220, then multiply that remaining number by 60 percent and 80 percent and you will have your range. I would strongly suggest staying at the 60 percent level and even less if your arm tends to swell when you exercise. It is important to wear either a support garment or bandages while exercising.

Be sure not to fatigue or overwork the muscles, as this can cause an increase in lymph fluid and make the lymphedema worse.[9] Normally, swimming, walking, and bike riding are very good exercise choices when you have lymphedema. Drs. John and Judith Casley-Smith found that scuba diving is also a wonderful activity for reduction of lymphedema, the effects lasting as long as two days.[10]

For regular swimming or pool exercise, many people find it helpful to wear an old support garment into the water. There are some especially good dance and yoga movements as well. Saskia Thiadens, R.N., president of the National Lymphedema Network, recommends a new videotape called *Focus on Healing Through Movement and Dance for the Breast Cancer Survivor.*[11]

No matter what exercise you choose, it is important to do only a small amount at first (just a few minutes if you haven't been a regular exerciser, and a bit more if you had a previously higher level of exercise), and then *gradually* increase the level of exercise over time, using your arm as a monitor of how much you can do. It is better not to exercise in the heat of the day, and be sure to protect yourself from the sun.

Choose a Light Prosthesis

If you have had a mastectomy and choose to wear a prosthesis, the National Lymphedema Network recommends wearing a light one. The weight of a heavy prosthesis may put too much pressure above the collarbone and increase the risk of interrupting the lymphatic flow.[1] There are also prostheses that are attached by adhesives on the skin. Many women who have these seem to love them and find them easier to wear than other types of prostheses they have tried. These might be recommended for some women, but if you use the adhesive, be very careful to avoid skin irritation.

Plan Ahead When You Travel

When you are at risk for developing lymphedema or already have it, traveling requires planning ahead and following some precautionary measures. First, when exploring your options for where to travel, consider how to make it easier on your lymph system (which doesn't like heat). Perhaps it would be better to pick a cooler season when you travel to a warmer climate. If you have a history of infection, it may be advisable to speak with your doctor about carrying a prescription for antibiotics with you.

If you are traveling by car, take frequent rest breaks and get out of your car and move around. Practice some simple mobility exercises for your neck, shoulders, and arm while you are in the car (specific exercise routines will be covered in a later chapter). Routinely practice abdominal breathing (discussed later), which will stimulate your central lymph trunks. Sit with a straight posture (sometimes a small pillow to support your low back helps with this). Avoid exposing your arm to sun, even through your car window.

If you are traveling by air, the change in cabin pressure when you are in flight may cause your arm to swell. Many women first notice their swelling during or after travel by air. It can help to wear a support garment if you have one, or to put on short stretch bandages (these will be discussed in a later chapter). If you are traveling long distances or for extended time periods, wear the bandaging over the support garment.[12] The same advice applies as in car travel: do some simple mobility exercises, practice diaphragmatic breathing, maintain good posture (ask the flight attendant to find one of those small airline pillows for you to support your back), and stand up and move around as much as you are allowed. Also, avoid caffeine and alcohol and drink lots of water.[1]

As previously advised, be careful when carrying heavy bags, especially with your arm straight down. Get a suitcase on wheels. Pack two smaller bags with less weight rather than one heavy one. Use the carts available in airports, or use porters. Check your bags at the curb if that service is available. Don't swing that carry-on bag over your affected shoulder.

Eat Healthful Foods

We like to refer to this as "eating style" rather than "diet." A diet is something you go on today and off tomorrow. Eating style is simply how you eat. Now is the time to create an eating style for yourself and your family that promotes optimal health for life. Ninety years of research have shown that what you eat is an important factor in the development and prevention of disease.[13] Our diet and our immune system are linked. Poor nutrition can significantly decrease immune function, and certain dietary modifications can enhance the immune system.[14] While there are no specific dietary guidelines or factors in the development of lymphedema, we recommend a healthy eating style.[15] Following are some general principles to observe.

◆ Eat plenty of fresh vegetables, fruits, whole grains, and legumes. These provide an abundance of fiber, vitamins, and minerals. Diets high in fiber have long been recognized for their role in preventing colon cancer and heart disease. Antioxidants in these foods are also thought to help prevent cancer.[16]

◆ Eat a moderate amount of protein from beans and bean products such as tofu and lentils. Incorporate a number of seeds, nuts, and fish in your diet, and de-emphasize meats, poultry, and eggs. While it might seem logical to reduce protein intake, since lymphedema is a high-protein edema, it is absolutely necessary to have sufficient protein. Eating too little protein will not reduce the protein content in the lymph fluid, but it will weaken the connective tissue and worsen the lymphedema.[17]

◆ Try to minimize the fat in your diet. High-fat diets have been associated with cancer of the colon and breast. The recommendation by nutritionists is to reduce the level of saturated fat intake by two-thirds.[18] However, keep in mind that some fats are essential to health. The fat in fish has been shown to enhance the clearance of dietary fat and to lessen the blood's tendency to form clots. The recommendation is to eat fish twice a week.[16]

◆ Wherever possible, eat foods in their natural rather than processed form. For example, fresh vegetables have more food value than frozen vegetables, which have more food value than canned vegetables.

◆ Minimize your salt consumption. Salt can cause water retention.

❧ Minimize your intake of caffeine and alcohol. Excessive use of these fluids may contribute to fluid retention. (A side note unrelated to lymphedema: caffeine and alcohol also lead to excretion of calcium from the body, which can contribute to osteoporosis.) [16]

❧ A final recommendation: *increase* water consumption. Contrary to what might seem reasonable with lymphedema, where there is an excess of fluid, it is imperative to drink lots of water. The high-protein concentration of your arm attracts the fluid in your body. If you are taking in less water, it is not your arm that will have less fluid; it will be the rest of your body that is deprived of water. Drinking lots of water will also help to flush your system of impurities. It is recommended that you drink at least eight 8-ounce glasses of water a day.

We recommend any of the New American Diet cookbooks[16] by Dr. Sonja L. Connor, M.S., R.D., and William E. Connor, M.D., for excellent nutritional information, guidelines, and recipes. There are many other cookbooks containing excellent dietary advice. Check your local bookstore or library.

Summary

Until there is more research into what activities actually trigger lymphedema, and which help reduce it, we recommend that you take a practical, commonsense approach toward it all.[19]

Be kind to yourself. Keep in mind that, no matter how careful you might be, some lymphedema may not be preventable. You do not need to become obsessive (though if you're worried, it may be hard not to obsess). The point is to live even if you do have lymphedema. Attend to it, work its care into your daily habits so you can forget about it, and get back to living, working, and enjoying life.

Part Two

Treating Lymphedema

8

General Principles of Treatment

SOME OF US ARE FORTUNATE and may be able to prevent an episode of lymphedema. Others, however, will need treatment. This chapter gives an overview of the form that the most successful treatment takes.

In the beginning it is important to follow *all* recommended treatment modalities. The best results come from treating your lymphedema using all four of the processes outlined to the International Society of Lymphology in 1995 by Dr. Robert Lerner and already mentioned in chapter 6: massage, bandaging, exercise, and skin care. We have already addressed skin care in the chapter on prevention; the chapters that follow explore the other three processes.

Dr. Lerner's study, which followed one thousand patients with upper extremity lymphedema, is worth mentioning here again, as it points out the effectiveness of this high-intensity program. Using all four types of treatment at once, his patients experienced an average reduction of 62 percent in the volume of their lymphedema.[1] This is supported in a study published by Marvin Boris, M.D. and Bonnie B. Lasinski, P.T. in 1997, where they reported an average 63 percent reduction in the lymphedema volume in affected arms. Their study also showed that those patients who were most compliant in their follow-up care were able to maintain their initial reduction in volume and even improve it.[2]

In the later phases you can take more of a maintenance

approach, using those parts of treatment that help you most. Certainly, more consistent follow-through with the self-treatment of compression, exercise, and self-massage will more effectively manage the lymphedema.

We believe that most women will want to spend the least possible time balancing busy lives with the time it takes to get their symptoms under control. Also, the treatment is not a cookbook in which the same recipe works exactly the same for everyone. There is not an "only way," but simply "a way." Dr. Stephen Chandler reports feedback from patients who have received lymphedema treatment. "Not everybody," he says, "is helped by the treatments that are available." But he goes on to say, "All of my patients who have sought help have been gratified and have benefited in some way. Some people have time to devote to it and some don't; it is time-consuming. All who have had treatment for lymphedema have been pleased that someone knows how to help. The approaches women take to deal with lymphedema will benefit them the entire rest of their lives."

To a degree, philosophies and approaches may vary somewhat, but the basic focus is always the same: to reroute the fluid from the side of your body with the impaired lymphatic system and move it to an area of better drainage. What you will find in the following chapters is a compilation of Gwen's experience as well as a distillation of the work of people from all over the world who are experts on lymphedema.

Before we launch into a discussion of these techniques, there is one simple thing you can do right now on your own: elevate your arm. Elevation in the early stages is sometimes effective, using gravity to drain the fluid.[3] This has been one of the few suggestions doctors have offered in the past, and many people have gone to great lengths to keep their swollen limb up in the air. We suggest placing your arm on pillows while in bed, putting your arm over the back of the couch while watching TV or reading, and lying down during the day for short periods, if you are able, with your arm elevated over your body. When you are in the car, you can rest your arm on the car window ledge as long as you keep your arm covered to avoid exposure to the sun.

These simple measures may help decrease the swelling, particularly during the early onset of lymphedema, though in later stages elevation has little effect. However, elevation should not be your only course of action. If your arm is swollen, seek help. In the following chapters you will learn where to find a qualified health care practitioner who can help you, and you will learn many additional and very effective techniques to reduce the swelling in your arm. We suggest you earnestly try every technique we mention.

9

Lymphatic Massage: MLD®, or Manual Lymph Drainage

LYMPHATIC MASSAGE is a special form of very gentle massage that removes excess fluid and protein from an extremity with lymphedema and encourages the fluid to move into an area where it can drain away normally.

The massage starts with the trunk and other areas of your body not involved with lymphedema. The goal is to empty those areas first, clearing them to allow a place for the lymph fluid to drain to. Only then is the involved limb massaged.

On the involved limb, the massage starts with the area closest to the trunk and gradually moves farther down the limb: from the upper arm toward the hand, or down the leg to the foot.

The main physiological effects of lymphatic massage are to drain and cleanse the tissues in the body, to cause a relaxation response by stimulation of the parasympathetic part of the autonomic nervous system, and to provide pain relief.[1]

The term *manual lymph drainage* (MLD®) was coined by the Vodders and refers to this technique of lymphatic massage. Other practitioners have referred to it as "lymphatic mobilization." It is important to receive treatments from someone who has been thoroughly trained in lymph drainage massage. Other types of massage can cause an *increase* in fluid to the area. The therapist must have a complete understanding of the dynamics of lymphedema and its treatment.[2] See chapter 28, "Where to Get Help," if you wish to find clinics and therapists.

The therapist will use techniques that are gentle, slow, rhythmical, repetitive, circular, and light, and that employ a special pressure/release stroke.

Since the neck is near the end of the lymph system as it joins the venous system and then transports the lymph on to the heart, the massage begins there. The neck area is massaged to clear it of fluid and to stimulate the lymph angions (single lymph vessels), which, in turn, motivates them to contract. Research is currently under way to determine the total effect of MLD®. Preliminary results indicate that lymphatic massage of the neck area even stimulates activity of a lymph angion in the big toe![3]

The therapist then moves on to massage the *uninvolved* side of the body to stimulate the lymphatics to clear out fluid. The massage gradually moves to the involved side, then on to the involved limb. The light strokes are always in the direction of desired lymph flow. Massage of the abdominal area may be included to stimulate the deep lymphatic vessels.

As mentioned above, the arm massage starts with the shoulder and moves down the arm to the hand. The therapist will direct the massage pressure *toward* the direction in which the fluid should move. The massage should *never* be painful or cause reddening of the skin.

Different types of strokes are used depending on the area, type of tissue, integrity of the tissue, size of the area, and so on. Different sequences are used depending upon the type of cancer and surgery, whether there has been radiotherapy, and whether one or two sides of the body are involved. Usually the massage takes forty-five minutes to an hour. It can take longer if both the arms and the trunk are involved. The massage should be very soothing. People often fall asleep during a session.

When Should You *Not* Have a Massage?

There are times when it is advisable to not have lymphatic massage:[4]

♦ If you have active cancer. Theoretically, lymphatic massage could move cancer cells to a new area and potentially spread the cancer. However, this is a controversial topic. Others feel the risk of spreading cancer cells is so small it should not be a contraindication for lymphedema treatment. Discuss your situation with your doctor and therapist and decide what is best for you.

❖ If you have an infection. Signs of infection in the arm include redness, warmth to the touch, pain, and a sudden unexplained increase in swelling. After an effective course of antibiotics, when the infection is gone, massage can be resumed.

❖ If you have congestive heart failure. Lymphatic massage moves fluid out of the limb and through the body to the heart. In a person experiencing congestive heart failure there is already too much fluid around the heart. Doing lymphatic massage may have life-threatening consequences. There are some situations in which lymphatic massage might be done, but only with strict and close medical monitoring. Again, it is advisable to discuss your situation with your doctor and therapist.

❖ If you are being treated for thrombosis or blood clots. There is the potential with lymphatic massage to dislodge clots and allow them to move to the heart or lungs where they could be fatal. Massage must be avoided if you are being treated for this condition.

It is best to wait before working directly on fragile, irradiated skin. In such cases it is possible to do some modified massage, avoiding areas of fragile skin until they are healed.

Precautions

In order to design an appropriate treatment and exercise program for you, your therapist will probably ask for a thorough medical history, including your current symptoms. You may be questioned about your blood pressure, thyroid problems, chronic inflammation, asthma, and other health issues that may affect treatment.[5] Your therapist will want to take precautions if you suffer from some ailment such as kidney disease, diabetes, hypertension, asthma, or arterial disease. Your therapist may even obtain indications from your medical history that a comprehensive treatment program should not be provided.[6]

The lymphatic massage done by a therapist is just one piece of a total program to control lymphedema. In the next chapter you will begin to learn what you can do on your own to maintain and promote the reduction in swelling.

10

Self-Massage

SELF-MASSAGE IS LIKELY TO BECOME an integral part of your treatment program. We believe the work you can do for yourself supplements the treatment by the therapist and has long-term benefits. It gives you a tool to more effectively control the lymphedema and empowers you to treat yourself immediately when a therapist is not available. If you see your lymphedema start to increase, as it might during hot weather or when traveling on an airplane, you can take action to limit or eliminate a buildup.

As with the MLD® done by a therapist, when you self-massage you begin with your neck and trunk before going to the involved arm. It can be helpful to massage just the neck and trunk as this clears the way ahead and gives the limb a better chance of draining. In fact, the trunk massage is so important Gwen finds it best to stress it first so that patients do not, in their haste to reduce the swelling in their arm, move too fast to massaging the arm. If the arm alone is massaged, the fluid moves to the top of the arm, and if the trunk is not clear to receive the fluid, the fluid flows right back into the arm. The trunk and neck must be cleared first.

Gwen suggests that patients do the self-massage for the trunk before they wrap their arm in bandages and carry out the home exercise program.

Self-Massage Guidelines

What follows is one possible self-massage routine, though your therapist may suggest another routine. As with any treatment, it is important to work with a therapist who has been thoroughly trained in lymphedema treatment.

Make sure the area is free of oils, creams, or talcum powder so that your hands don't slide over the skin.

Use flat fingers or the palm of your hand. Do not push in with your fingertips. The massage requires two types of strokes: stationary circles, which are a circular motion in one spot, and sweeps, in which the skin is pushed gently in the direction the fluid is to flow. The massage stroke is very slow—each stroke should take at least one second to complete.

Apply just enough pressure to cause the skin to move slightly. The pressure in lymphatic massage should be very, very light.[1] The skin may wrinkle in front of your hand or finger movement and/or spring back when you lift your hand off the skin. The pressure must also be released with each stroke so the massage is a repetitive, pressure-on/pressure-off technique.

Massage strokes on the arm should be directed toward the outside of the arm and then up toward the body. Visualize moving the fluid away from your hand and toward your heart.

Massage should *never* cause pain or reddening of the skin.

Take deep abdominal breaths throughout your self-massage (see chapter 19, "Breathing Exercises"), inhaling through your nose and relaxing the abdomen as it fills with air, then exhaling through pursed lips as you pull in your stomach muscles and the abdomen contracts.

Self-Massage for Upper Extremity Lymphedema

Start with an abdominal breathing exercise. Whenever stationary circles are recommended, they should be repeated twenty times. All sweep motions should be repeated five to seven times (see Figures 10-1 and 10-2).

1. Massage your neck (Figure 10-1) using stationary circles with your hands crossed. Make small, coin-sized circles, pumping down and releasing up in the hollow above both collarbones.

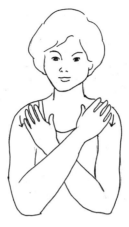

Figure 10-1. Self-lymphatic-massage for the neck

2. Pump up and release down with stationary circles in the armpit on the uninvolved side.

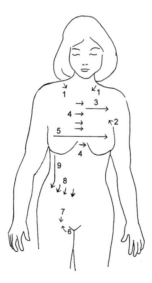

Figure 10-2. Self-lymphatic-massage for right-arm lymphedema

3. Sweep skin from the midline (vertical watershed) of the chest toward the uninvolved armpit. Do this in several places along chest.

4. Sweep skin across the midline watershed, moving down the chest from neck to navel.

5. Sweep skin from the involved armpit across to the uninvolved armpit. Repeat several times across the chest wall. Go around scars.

6. Pump up and release down using stationary circles in the groin on the involved side.

7. Sweep skin from the horizontal watershed to the groin.

8. Sweep skin over the horizontal watershed.

9. Sweep skin from the armpit on the involved side down to the groin.

Repeat #1.

Self-Massage Especially for the Arm

As mentioned before, the arm should never be massaged until *after* the neck and trunk have been massaged. Repeat each sweep five to seven times. Stationary circles can be done fifteen to twenty times (see Figures 10-3 and 10-4).

Upper Arm

1. Sweep skin up on the outside of your arm, around the back of your shoulder, and into the nodes above your collarbone.

2. Sweep skin on your upper arm inside to outside up to the back of your shoulder (sweep in three different places along the upper arm from armpit to elbow). Do the front of the upper arm first, then the back of the upper arm.

Elbow

3. Pump up and release down in stationary circles at the bend of your elbow. Your massage stroke should be directed to the outer part of your arm.

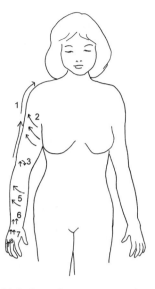

Figure 10-3. Lymphatic massage for right arm

4. If fibrosis (thickening) is present around the elbow, pump up and release down a little more firmly. As the tissue softens, move to the next area around the elbow.

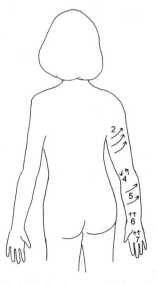

Figure 10-4. Lymphatic massage for right arm

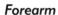

Forearm

5. Sweep skin up on the inside and outside of your forearm.

Wrist

6. Pump up and release down in stationary circles or use a sweep motion up around the wrist. Increase the pressure a little if fibrosis is present.

Hand

7. Pump up and release down in stationary circles or use a sweep motion on the palm and back of your hand.

   Sweep skin on your fingers and thumb toward the back of your hand.

   Finish by raising your arm overhead. Sweep skin from your fingertips down the back of your hand, wrist, and forearm to the outside of your upper arm, the back of your shoulder, and finally, down your side to the groin area.

Back Massage by a Partner

While you can do most of the massage yourself, it can be helpful (as well as relaxing) to have someone else do it for you. This is especially helpful when doing lymphatic massage to the back, where it is very awkward and not really advisable to massage yourself. Stimulating the back with lymphatic massage provides another alternative drainage pathway across the watershed that runs vertically down the middle of your back. The techniques and strokes should follow the same guidelines as when you are doing it yourself.

This can be done as a part of the trunk massage, but before doing the arm massage. You can sit leaning over a table with pillows for support, arms reaching forward, and your forehead resting on your hands. An alternative position is to lie on your stomach with your arms at your side, forehead resting on a rolled towel or small pillow.

Remind your partner to use very light, slow pressure and to always release the pressure with each stroke. Practice deep breathing while you are having the massage. Inhale through your nose and relax the abdomen as it fills with air. Exhale through pursed lips.

Here is the technique see (Figure 10-5):

1. Pump up and release down in stationary circles at both armpits. Do twenty repetitions.

2. Sweep skin from the vertical watershed toward the uninvolved armpit in several places.

3. Sweep skin across the vertical watershed in several places along spine.

4. Sweep skin from the involved armpit across to the uninvolved armpit in several places.

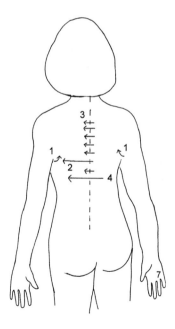

Figure 10-5. Back lymphatic massage

Note from Jeannie: For me, self-massage is the treatment I have continued (along with occasional bandaging), even after my lymphedema subsided. I usually take a few minutes for it two or three times a week.

At first, while I was just learning self-massage, I worked very hard to emulate the techniques Gwen used while she massaged me. I tried to duplicate the pressure she applied, and to copy the types of strokes she used, unless there was some area that had become harder (fibrotic); then I dug in with a little more pressure until it softened. I even weighed my own fingers' pressure on a postage meter—it was just six ounces.

As I went along, I grew frustrated I couldn't do much to massage my own back. Then I figured out something that seemed to help. (Keep in mind, this is my idea, not something Gwen or any doctor would prescribe.)

I bought a new paint roller with a super-fluffy sheath (the kind for real rough walls), and I learned to use it on my back. I roll from my ribs across my back and along my shoulder to apply pressure in ways I couldn't manage without it.

Do I feel silly using my paint roller? You bet. But it seems to help, even if the benefit is only in my mind.

If you try this trick, the lightest ones are the easiest to use, and make sure you get one that doesn't squeak!

❖ ❖ ❖

Self-massage is an important component of managing lymphedema. In the next chapter, meet D.J. Self-massage has been important in keeping her lymphedema at bay.

11

D.J.: An Athlete Uses Self-Massage

IT IS SEVEN O'CLOCK AT NIGHT and we are meeting for dinner at a restaurant in the neighborhood near D.J.'s house.

On the telephone, D.J. told me she's thirty-nine but added, "I still get carded when I buy liquor." She described herself as "five-eight, with short hair shaved on the sides. Sometimes I'm mistaken for a guy."

She enters the restaurant wearing a pair of huge jeans cut off at the knees, a silver chain changing from her belt, and a T-shirt decorated with an amazing and beautiful picture of a tiger. Without saying a word, she ducks her head in greeting and sits down.

She begins relating her story. "My mother died of ovarian cancer," she says, "when she was fifty. By the time they discovered it, my mother was too far gone for surgery. They gave her radiation and chemotherapy, but I think it just weakened her. She spent the last six months of her life in a hospital."

There is no sense of loss or sadness as D.J. says this, but there is an aspect to her face that says she has come to grips with it and is now relating it because her own history demands the telling. She continues in a kind of stride, starting on the story of her own cancer and how she discovered a lump in her breast. "It was a real weird time," she says. "I had just been evicted from the apartment where I lived for eight years—the building sold and the new owner wanted to live in my apartment. A day later I discovered the lump. On top of everything else, I had just

63

changed health insurance companies, and I didn't know any doctors at the new place. I had a mammogram. The radiation technologist showed me the film, said she was pretty sure what we were seeing was cancer. Well, it turned out it was a tumor.

"I have to admit that the surgeon seemed to be treating me well. I'm gay. Sometimes that causes people to act in odd ways. It's hard as a gay person to trust doctors. But he didn't seem disrespectful. He even seemed at ease with my partner and all her questions. But I wanted a double mastectomy. He refused to do it. I had no doubts. And as hard as I insisted, he resisted, saying my medical coverage wouldn't cover it. I said I was willing to pay by myself, and I was starting to let him know I was going to get another surgeon. He finally relented. I have never regretted my decision. Not once."

There were no lymph nodes removed, she says, and she was not scheduled for chemotherapy or radiation. She thought she was over the episode of cancer, and she and her partner bought a house together. Six months later she had plastic surgery to smooth over some irregularities in her scars. She noticed another lump after the plastic surgery. "It turned out to be a recurrence. The needle biopsy showed it was positive."

The surgeons removed the lump, but the margins weren't clear. It was a highly aggressive, fast-growing tumor situated between two layers of muscle. "This time, they gave me chemotherapy and radiation." Because she is premenopausal, she decided not to take Tamoxifen.

Not long after her radiation treatments, she began experiencing problems with lymphedema. "It wasn't swelling so much," she says, "but I was getting numbness." She lifts her arm, strokes under the upper part of it. "It was numb along here," she says. "I knew I'd get it here. But it started getting numb down on the lower part as well, and in my fingers." She spreads the fingers on her right hand. "I couldn't even do this," she says.

"I guess because I'm into computers," she smiles, "I went online. I found out all kinds of ugly things about lymphedema—that it wasn't curable, that it was deforming, that doctors didn't care about it if it wasn't killing you. Everything I found terrified me. The thing I was most afraid of wasn't a recurrence of cancer, but the lymphedema.

"I'm real athletic. I play town-team softball. I thought I'd have to give it up. I thought I was going to have to give up painting my house. Here I had bought myself a house and I couldn't even paint. I panicked when I thought it was going to change my life.

"One of the hardest things was I didn't think I could get a tattoo. I really want this special tattoo I've designed with cats and tigers running across my chest. This tattoo is real important to me." The smile disappeared. "But I don't think I can risk it now." She looks down, begins idly playing with her spoon. "All those little needle pricks might lead to more of the lymphedema," she says.

She looks up again, puts her hand in her lap. "Anyway, I was referred to a physical therapist, and I had one appointment before a softball tournament last summer. I went ahead and played ball, but I couldn't hit anything. My hand just didn't work right." She spreads her fingers again. "It's a lot better now, but the weather's not hot any more, either. I wonder what it will be like next summer."

She says she doesn't do any of the self-treatments of bandaging or wearing compression garments. "But I do the self-massage," she says. "So far, it's what I am willing to do. It does seem to help. And I do some exercises with a squeeze ball to keep circulation in my hand. I don't know if I'm going to be able to play softball next year. I am starting to go to the gym to work out. I'm just going to have to wait and see how much it's going to change my life.

"People live with lymphedema. It isn't a death sentence. Life may be changed by it, but life doesn't have to end because of it."

12

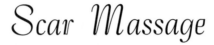

Scar Massage

Besides self-massage to manage lymphedema, you may want to consider massage to the scar tissue that develops after surgery. In fact, this self-treatment of the scar area is important whether or not you have lymphedema.

Scar massage mobilizes your scar and restores normal mobility of the skin and underlying tissues following your mastectomy or lumpectomy. You may begin massaging the scar when it is well healed (when all the scabs have fallen off naturally).

This massage differs from lymphatic massage in the amount of pressure you want to apply. The benefit from massage to a scar is greatest when the skin is worked as firmly as possible, just below your pain threshold. Be sure to start gently and progress to a deeper and stronger massage—you should never cause yourself sharp, stabbing pain. However, it is common to have slight discomfort, such as a pulling or a light burning sensation, during the massage.

Here is the technique:

Set aside five minutes a day to perform scar massage. Include all your scars, even the ones in your armpit. You may find it easier to do this massage while facing a mirror. To begin, place your hand (on the operated side) on the top of your head.

Use the pads of two or three fingers held together, slightly arched, and keep them on the area you are massaging. Don't slide across the skin.

Do not use lotion or oil during the massage, because it will cause your fingers to slide around. You need to affect the deeper tissues under the skin and must use firm pressure. Apply lotion to the area *after* the massage. Vitamin E is especially good for the skin and for scars.

Start with a light pressure and then progress to a firmer stroke. You may notice one or two directions that feel "stuck." Spend a little more time in those areas.

Now, the actual massage:

1. Using one hand, massage parallel to the scar on each side, repeating this three to five times. Then move on to the next section of skin until you have covered the entire incision area.

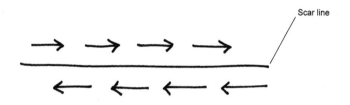

Figure 12-1. Scar massage (a)

2. Using one hand, make circular strokes in a similar fashion, both clockwise and counterclockwise, across the top of the scar and just below the scar.

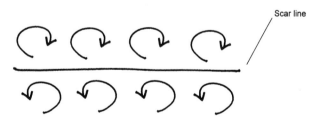

Figure 12-2. Scar massage (b)

Massage After Radiotherapy

After you have completed radiotherapy, you may need to do some deeper scar massage over the irradiated tissue if it is tight and bound down. Wait until the skin is well healed from radiotherapy before beginning any massage. The same techniques work for radiation scar tissue as for the incision scar. Be sure to apply lotion or oil after the massage.

Because scar tissue can develop up to six months after radio-therapy has been completed, it is important to continue checking the skin for hardness, thickening, or binding down in the areas that have been irradiated.

❖ ❖ ❖

Although the discussion in this chapter does not pertain directly to lymphedema, it points out the need to restore tissue to health once it has been treated. It is worth doing anything we can to help our bodies heal and to reduce the chances for problems later on, not just in our arms but anywhere in our bodies.

Linda's story in the next chapter highlights a case of lymphedema settling in the trunk of the body after breast cancer treatment. She tells of coming up with a creative way to work the scar tissue that developed after her surgery.

13

Linda: Massaging Scars and Dealing with Lymphedema of the Torso

LINDA HAS COME TO THE MEDICAL FACILITY to be treated for lymphedema. She has squeezed our interview into the time between her physical therapy exercise and her appointment with the therapist for lymph treatment.

We are sitting at a table in the cafeteria of the medical facility. Linda is wearing casual clothes; a plaid snap-button shirt and jeans. She is of medium height and build, and is neat, though her shirt is not tucked into her jeans.

Linda is in her mid-forties. Her children still live at home, though they are almost grown. She says she has been living with her fiancé, Ron, for seven years. She is a thoughtful woman. There is the sense she would never utter an unplanned word.

"Before I met Ron, I worked at a large corporation. I started out as an executive secretary. They promoted me to inventory and dispatching the fleet, but that didn't work out, so I quit and I'm working with my fiancé managing a KOA campground.

"My mother had cancer eleven years ago," Linda says. "She went through surgery, chemotherapy, and radiotherapy, but despite all that work, the cancer spread to her bones. Two years after my mother died, I found out I had cancer."

"I was luckier than my mother," she says with a bit of sarcasm. "They found my cancer before it had spread to my lymph nodes. I didn't have to have chemotherapy."

Then, just a year ago, Linda found out she had cancer again, in the other breast. "I never felt a lump," she says. She had a mastectomy. "But the surgery didn't go well at all." Her lips gather in as if she is momentarily dealing with some anger. "Somehow they pulled a wrong tube, and a couple of days later I started to swell. I learned later the swelling was lymphedema. Then it became infected. Everything went wrong. I reacted to the antibiotics and spent four days in the hospital.

"After I was released, the infection came back. I was in the hospital five days the second time. The swelling was terrible. And when I finally went home, I had to keep going back two and three times a week to have them aspirate the swelling. Each time, the doctor removed anywhere from a few drops of fluid to as much as a cup or two cups.

"That went on for six weeks. I was commuting seven and eight hundred miles a week. It was awful."

The swelling did not subside. It manifested in her torso. "It's still there," she says. She leans back, pulls at her shirt, and indicates a handful of flesh. "See?" She moves her hands to the other side, where there is much less bulk. "And it's down from what it used to be.

"Nobody seemed to know anything about lymphedema. Even what little information the doctor gave me only mentioned it occurring in arms and legs.

"I didn't know what to do until I went to a physical therapist for problems I was having with my jaw. They thought I might have TMJ." She shakes her head. "I was also developing a spinal problem because of the dramatic changes in my sitting and sleeping posture.

"When I went to the physical therapist for TMJ treatment, she said she thought lymphedema was a more significant problem than anything else and she began treating me for that. She thought the weight of the imbalance was throwing my posture off."

Linda continues, "I've been coming into town for lymphedema treatment one and two times a week for the last five months. It's getting a little better. And some time ago I started taking medication for depression. My energy is a little better.

"I have started working out on an exercise bicycle, and three times a week I'm doing the self-massage the therapist taught me and I work some on the scars." Almost as an afterthought she says, "And I use a massager."

As we talk further about the massager, she becomes more animated. The idea of using it came to her on her own. It seems to capture an intense expression of hope. "It's in my purse," she says. She brings out something that looks like a flashlight with a rounded top about the size of a showerhead.

Linda strokes the smooth head of the massager. "It takes three batteries," she says. She flips a switch on the side of it. It hums to life. She makes a motion toward her waist, where she has the most swelling. "I run it between my ribs," she says. "I think it helps."

A few weeks after our interview, we communicate again on the Internet. The tone of her note is hopeful. "Between the treatments I have been having and the massage thing I bought, the bag of fluid on my belly is gone. The massager does all the work for me. I just have to move it around to hit all the right spots. Spending extra time directly on the hard scar tissue seems to be beneficial, too. I don't plan to feel like a sloppy, fat couch potato for much longer."

14

Compression Using Bandages

COMPRESSING TISSUE THAT IS SWOLLEN is another aspect of lymphedema treatment. In this chapter we discuss bandages, and in the next chapter we look at various special compression garments you can purchase, which are often covered by insurance.

The bandages used are rolls of short-stretch cloth bandages that are wrapped around the involved extremity. Although they resemble sports bandages (ace wraps), which you are probably familiar with, they are not as stretchy. Do *not* try substituting sports bandages for them.

Compression bandages apply external pressure to a swollen limb. When swelling has persisted in an area, the tissue loses some of its elasticity and does not return to its original position and shape even when the fluid decreases. The bandages support the skin and its underlying vessels.

Bandaging normally starts with a white gauze wrap at the fingers and then continues with a series of different-sized short-stretch bandages around the hand, progressing up the arm to within a short distance of the shoulder. The number of bandages used depends on the size of the arm and how effectively the compression is achieved, but usually at least three bandages are necessary.

Never wrap bandages tightly, just pull enough to take up the slack and roll the bandages onto the arm. The amount of compression is determined by how many layers of bandages are applied. The compression should be even throughout the arm, and if the compression varies in an area (it feels looser and then tighter) another bandage is used in that area to even up the pressure.

By using external support bandages, you can enhance other phases of treatment and ensure their success.[1] Bandaging helps by:

◈ Creating a semirigid support for the muscle to work against, improving the muscle pumping action, and causing a movement of lymph fluid.[2]

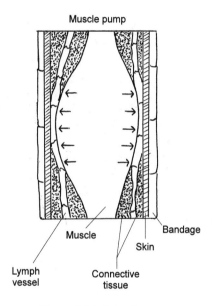

Muscle pump

Muscle   Bandage

Skin

Lymph vessel   Connective tissue

Figure 14-1. Muscle pump

◈ Influencing movement of fluid in the tissue channels, causing interstitial fluid to move into the functioning lymph system.

◈ Increasing total tissue pressure, which causes venous capillaries and the initial lymph vessels to take in more fluid and causes arterial capillaries to release less fluid.[2] The circulatory system decreases the amount of fluid it sends into the tissues and increases the ability of the veins to pull fluid back into the vessels.

◈ Improving and maintaining the shape of the arm. When

someone is going through a comprehensive lymphedema treatment regimen, the size of the arm is most likely changing. The bandage keeps the amount of compression consistent with that change and helps to reshape the limb.[3]

Why Can't I Use Ace Wraps, Which Are Much Less Expensive?

Sports bandages, such as Ace wraps, are high-stretch elastic bandages and are not effective in treating lymphedema. When your muscles are at rest, the constant compression of the sports bandage does not allow the lymphatic vessels to fill and thereby prevents draining of fluid from the tissue. When your muscles contract, the sports bandage is so stretchy that it does not provide a rigid enough support for them to pump against. This kind of bandaging does not raise tissue pressure enough to effectively influence the lymphatic pump.[2]

Principles of Compression Bandaging

Here are some guidelines that help ensure success in bandaging:

* Greater pressure should be applied to the hand and lower forearm, with a gradual reduction in pressure moving proximally up the limb toward the trunk. This is done not by applying bandages tighter at the hand and forearm but by having a greater number of layers and overlap of bandages.[2] The width of the bandages will vary depending on the circumference of the arm. (Bandages come in widths of six, eight, ten, and twelve centimeters; 5 centimeters = 2 inches.) The number of bandages will vary with the size and shape of the arm and the person's tolerance. Normally the fingers are wrapped with one-inch and two-inch gauze bandages.

* Appropriate padding is necessary to protect the skin and bony prominences, and to provide even distribution of the pressure over the entire limb. It also prevents chafing and

protects tender areas. A soft roll of cotton padding called Artiflex is available and made for this protection.

◆ Foam padding may be applied in order to shape the limb, or denser foam used to break down fibrotic areas. Different densities of foam may be cut into small pieces and placed in a small "chip" bag (Dr. Vodder's School calls these "chocolates"), which can be placed over areas of fibrosis or hardening.

◆ There is now available a "Legacy" compression sleeve designed by an experienced lymphedema therapist, JoAnn Rovig, CLT. It consists of a soft cloth sleeve of "chips," or foam pieces, sewn in a pattern designed to break up fibrosis and to assist directional lymph flow.[4] It can be used under bandaging or can also be worn while using a vasopneumatic pump. While there is no research as yet that quantitatively supports the sleeve's effectiveness, many patients and therapists report a rapid softening of hard areas of fibrosis with increased reduction in swelling.

◆ Fingers should be wrapped separately in gauze bandages.[3]

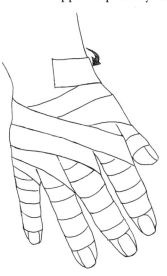

Figures 14-2. Finger wraps

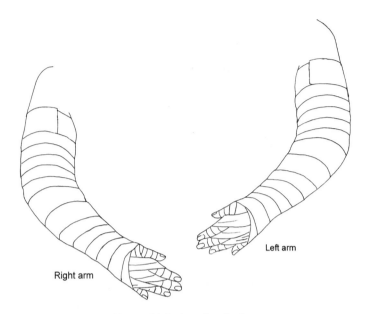

Right arm

Left arm

Figure 14-3. Arm bandaging

When Should You Bandage?

When you bandage may vary depending on the therapist you are seeing, where the therapist received training, how much treatment you have already received, how your arm is responding, and whether you have a support garment (discussed later). You should not try to bandage yourself until you have been instructed by a therapist specially trained in bandaging and lymphatic massage. If done improperly, bandaging can cause fluid buildup in the wrong areas or cause constriction, blocking the flow of fluid.

Most therapists will recommend you wear the bandages twenty-four hours a day in the intense phase of therapy, only taking them off to bathe and have treatment.[5] After your treatment is completed and you have a support garment, you may be able to gradually discontinue use of the bandages.

Other therapists suggest wearing the bandages while you sleep, as well as any time you are exercising or performing physical activity. Some suggest wearing them also after you have had lymphatic massage.[6]

After going through lymphedema treatment successfully, some patients simply use the bandages while exercising or to reduce the size of their arm during episodes of swelling. Many wear bandages at times when they may be at higher risk and swelling may be greater, such as in the summer, or when traveling by air (see chapter 7, "What Can I Do to Prevent Lymphedema?").

Some patients feel that since elevation helps with the swelling, it is safe to remove their bandages and/or garments when they sleep. This is actually a time when the bandaging can be most helpful, since in sleep the muscular action decreases and its pumping influence to the lymph vessels is diminished. This may cause the lymph fluid to pool and not move through the lymph system.[7]

It is probably a good idea to experiment. See what works best for you, and what is realistic for your lifestyle. Certainly the more you wear the bandages, the better the results will be. However, we know that, realistically, many people simply cannot or will not wear bandages twenty-four hours a day, yet they too can achieve some benefit. Many people are happy to see even small or moderate reductions and find this satisfactory even if their arm is not absolutely perfect. However long you wear them, bandages will give you some results, and this is better than if you never wear them at all.

Many women are satisfied simply knowing they can choose to do more to decrease the swelling in their arm, but they don't have to. Everyone has her own situation and needs to find what works best for her.

When Should You *Not* Bandage?

There are times when bandaging is not recommended, even if you are experiencing swelling:

- ❖ If you have an active infection in the arm. You should temporarily discontinue bandaging until the infection is under control. If you have any open wounds it is important to have them properly dressed, then to apply short-stretch bandages over them. This should be done only under medical supervision and may actually help with wound healing.

- If you have circulatory problems, nerve problems, or arterial insufficiency problems.

- If you feel pain. Although the bandages are not likely to be the most comfortable things you have ever experienced, they should not cause any level of significant pain or numbness in your arm. If they do cause pain, discontinue wrapping until you can discuss it with your therapist or doctor. Before removing the bandages, however, try going through the simple lymph drainage exercises in chapter 21 to see if the pain or numbness diminishes with movement.

- If you have a recurrence of cancer it is best to discontinue bandaging until you can discuss it with your doctor. Generally, with active cancer the recommendation is to discontinue massage techniques and bandaging, both of which actively move lymph fluid and theoretically could move cancer cells to other areas of your body. However, Drs. Judith Casley-Smith and the Foeldis feel cancer is not spread by this treatment. Dr. Casley-Smith does suggest that the bandages may be too uncomfortable or the patient may be too tired to bandage correctly. As there is controversy on this matter, it is advisable to discuss it with your doctor and therapist.

Care of Bandages

We suggest putting the bandages in net laundry bags used for socks or underclothing and washing them with a mild detergent on a gentle cycle in lukewarm water. They will last longer if they are laid out flat and air-dried; however, they can be put in the dryer on the gentle cycle. Launder them at least weekly or more frequently if they become soiled or soaked with perspiration.

Note from Jeannie: Because lymphedema was so frightening to me, I found it difficult to resume my normal life. Everything seemed to pose the possibility of making it worse.

But slowly, as I experimented, confidence came back to me as I added activities, sometimes holding my breath, then saw the effects they had on my swelling. Though I no longer need to bandage every day, as I did at the start of treatment, I still wrap when I'm going to be doing something strenuous like cleaning the house or gardening. I have a set of bandages that is stained green from the day I put in geraniums and is splattered with off-white Latex from painting the kitchen.

So far—knock wood—hard work doesn't seem to hurt me. In fact, if I bandage, my arm seems to benefit from a day of heavy effort.

I don't think there's any activity I can't do any more because of swelling, but I do take the precautions Gwen mentions throughout the book.

15

Compression with Special Garments

SINCE THE ELASTIC FIBERS OF THE SKIN are damaged by lymphedema, it is very important to apply sufficient compression in order to prevent the fluid from reaccumulating.[1] In the first, intense phases of treatment, compression is normally achieved by application of the short-stretch bandages. After the affected extremity has decreased in size, most patients should be fitted with a compression garment (sleeve) that is worn during the daytime. These garments are less bulky under clothing and are usually more comfortable than the bandages. The garments are not designed to reduce swelling, however, but to maintain the size of the limb and to prevent swelling from increasing.[2] For optimal ongoing lymphedema management, consistent and long-term use of compression garments is encouraged.[3] Some therapists are even recommending that patients wear the garment at night as well as during the day.

There are several things to consider when getting a garment. The time to get it is when treatment for lymphedema has been completed and the size of the arm has become fairly stable.[4] I suggest trying to fit into ready-made stock sizes first. These are not only less expensive but also take less time to get and require only three to four measurements. Custom garments are available if you do not fit a standard size. These require many measurements, cost two to three times more than stock sizes, and can take up to several weeks to be delivered. They are indicated, however, if the arm—or the leg, in cases of lower extremity lymphedema—does not fit into the size range of the standard garments or is awkwardly shaped.[5] The garment should provide the optimal compression without cutting in anywhere, and a custom-made garment may be necessary to accomplish that.[6]

There are different styles of garments, and the style you should get depends on your needs and the distribution of the swelling. There is a sleeve style that fits from the wrist to the armpit, and another that fits from the wrist to the top of the shoulder with a body strap. Most people also usually need a gauntlet (a garment for the hand). These also come in several different styles: one type covers just the palm and back of the hand and includes a partial thumb covering, but leaves the fingers free; another has the palm and back of the hand covered, as well as partial coverings for all the fingers; and the third type is like a full glove. The gauntlets can be either attached to the sleeve or worn separately (see Figure 15-1).

Other factors therapists take into consideration when preparing patients to obtain garments are the patient's age, independence, dexterity, and lifestyle, and even environmental factors such as climate.[7]

If you have trouble with the sleeve slipping down your arm, you might want to consider a shoulder flap, although, as Nancy mentions in her story in the next chapter, some manufacturers now have a silicone band, or beads, at the top of garments, which are designed to stick better to the skin in order to hold the garment up. Many patients have reported that these work very well and are easier to wear than the shoulder strap with its flaps. However, for some women, this silicone ring can cause a tourniquet effect. There is also body glue that some people find helpful in preventing the sleeve from slipping down. This can be obtained at medical supply companies that sell garments.

What will work best for you depends on the distribution of your swelling—and it is important to simply notice how your arm responds to the style you choose. Remember that the garment is an essential component of treatment, so it is crucial that it fit correctly.

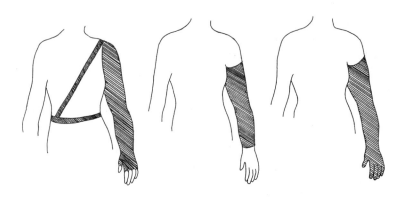

Figure 15-1. Arm compression garments

Several manufacturers in the United States make compression garments, and these will often be available at your local medical supply company. But to get the right fit, be sure to have someone helping you who is familiar with compression garments, ideally a certified fitter. In many cases, the therapist you are working with for decongestive lymphatic therapy will be able to measure you or guide you on where to go. There is a list of manufacturers of compression garments at the end of this chapter.

As we said, the garments come in a variety of styles. Even the fabrics differ. Options are available for sensitive skin, in lighter weight for summer, of various durabilities, and in different colors. Garments may be seamed or seamless. Seamless ones are knitted in the round and are usually preferred if they are available. They may be more comfortable than seamed garments, which makes them easier to wear.

Garments also differ in levels of compression. The most common level of compression sleeves is 20–40 mm Hg (leg garments may need to have a greater pressure). A lighter pressure is used if a person is wearing the garment twenty-four hours a day and is sleeping in it (which is rare) or if the recommended pressure for the garment is simply not tolerated.[7] If the lymphedema is severe, you may require a greater pressure of 40–50 mm Hg.

Patient Guidelines

Compression garments are generally worn under your clothing from the time you wake up until bedtime. (If you are bandaging at night, you will remove your garment in the early evening and apply bandages until the morning.) Garments are rarely worn at night, although an increasing number of therapists are recommending this.

Garments should be replaced when they are too tight, too loose, baggy due to age, or losing the ability to prevent limb refilling. Those patients bandaging at night can expect continuous gradual reductions and a possible change in size within two months. With light wear and tear, the garments may last as much as six months, but they often need to be replaced sooner than that.

A heavier garment made by the Jobst company and called an ELVAREX sleeve lasts longer but it is also significantly more expensive. It is suggested that you have two garments at any given time and alternate their use on a daily basis. Don't order the second garment until you are certain that the first fits well.

The garment should feel firm and supportive, *not painful*, and should not make the fingers turn a dusky purple or blue color. If you experience aching in the swollen arm after a period of inactivity, try moving around and exercising the limb rather than removing the sleeve. The discomfort may be due to a buildup of fluid and may decrease once you are active. If a tight band of constriction occurs, it may be a sign of a poorly fitting garment. A garment that does not fit well can actually contribute to more swelling and can be harmful to your arm.[8] Consult your therapist if any problems arise.

Application and Removal of Garments

While you will most likely feel awkward the first few times you put on the garment, with practice it does get easier. Here are some guidelines and suggestions that should help:

◆ Turn the arm sleeve partly inside out to initially place it on your arm.

- Use a rubber glove and/or powder to assist in putting on your compression garment. Use of the gloves also prevents expensive runs. Move the fabric up the arm bit by bit by gripping it with the rubber glove.

- Apply and remove the garment carefully to preserve the elasticity and life of the garment.

- Take care to make sure the garment is smooth, without wrinkles or folds, and the fabric is distributed evenly across the limb. Wrinkles can irritate your skin, or worse, act like elastic bands and cause fluid to build up beyond them.[8]

- Apply your compression garment when you first get up in the morning. If you wait until later in the morning, your arm may swell and the garment may not fit properly. Avoid putting it on directly after a bath—the moist skin and slightly increased swelling will make it a struggle.

- Check the garment throughout the day and pull up the sleeve if it slides down. You can use skin adhesive to help the garment stay up.

- You can remove the garment by grabbing the top and pulling it down over the limb so that it ends up inside out.

- Avoid using lotion under your garment unless it is a medical ointment or unless the manufacturer specifically says that you can use salves, lotions, or oils. There is a silicone-based lotion specifically designed to use under garments that keeps moisture in and doesn't damage the garment. Check with the garment manufacturer. Use your moisturizing lotions at night.

Laundering and Care of the Garment

Hand- or machine-wash your garment, on a gentle cycle, using a mild soap. Do not use Woolite. Launder the garment as you would any fine lingerie. Avoid bleach or fabric softeners. Rinse your hand-washed garment well. Roll or pat your garment dry in a towel. Do not twist it. Some brands of garments can be dried by machine using wash-and-wear settings.[9] Other manufacturers suggest you air-dry your garment.

A clean garment will last longer. Skin oils and dirt buildup will break down the resilience of the garment fibers. Wearing gloves or protective clothing over your garment when performing some indoor and outdoor activities may help keep your garment clean.

Manufacturers of Compression Garments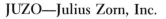

JUZO—Julius Zorn, Inc.
80 Chart Road, P.O. Box 1088
Cuyahoga Falls, OH 44223   Tel. (800) 222-4999

Medi USA
76 West Seegers Road
Arlington Heights, IL 60005   Tel. (800) 633-6334

Sigvaris, Inc.
P.O. Box 570
Branford, CT 06405   Tel. (800) 322-7744

Beiersdorf-Jobst
653 Miami St.
Toledo, OH 43694   Tel. (800) 537-1063

Gottfried Medical, Inc.
P.O. Box 8966
Toledo, OH 43623   Tel. (800) 537-1968

Bauerfeind USA
55 Chastain Road #112
Kennesaw, GA 30144   Tel. (800) 772-4534

Compression garments are now also available over the Internet. We have no personal experience with this method of finding them however and we recommend caution. It is very difficult to measure and apply a garment by yourself if you have never worn one before. And since a poorly fitting garment can worsen lymphedema, evaluate your situation carefully before using this do-it-yourself method, especially if it is your first garment.

◆ ◆ ◆

In the next chapter, Nancy details her experience with several different types of compression.

16

Nancy: A Nurse Uses Compression to Treat Her Lymphedema

NANCY IS A NURSE in Radiation Oncology. We are meeting at her clinic, where she is working our interview into her Friday afternoon schedule. Nancy told me she is forty, but her complexion has the freshness of an undergraduate. Her eyes are light blue and bright, and her skin is clear, her cheeks high-colored rose. She is wearing a nurse's sensible shoes and a clinical blue tunic with drawstring slacks. Over her tunic she wears a sweater.

She tells me first about her cancer diagnosis four years ago. "I knew right from the start," she says, "that I had cancer. I found a lump and just knew it right away.

"I went in for a mammogram. The cancer didn't show on it, but the lymph nodes were bright as neon." She has a professional's clear way of speaking, as if this were something that had happened to a patient of hers. "There was no history of breast cancer in my family, so it was not something that had been on my mind.

"The surgeon aspirated both the tumor and the nodes because the nodes were palpable. It turned out that, because I had stage II cancer and because all eleven lymph nodes the surgeon removed were positive for it, my prognosis was poor."

She became part of a clinical trial on high-dose chemotherapy and donated her own bone marrow for later transplant. Her treatments started with four months of chemotherapy, followed by high-dose chemotherapy. She was in the hospital for twenty-one days.

Seven months later, after chemotherapy, she started treatments with radiation. "Because of my prognosis, four fields— pretty much the maximum—were radiated."

Nancy gives a little personal background. She has been an RN almost twenty years. She is married, has a son, thirteen, and a daughter, fifteen. She started her nursing career in Intensive Care.

"But the hospital was a thirty- to forty-five-minute commute from home, so, after my treatment for cancer, I started thinking about a change to be nearer home. And by chance there was this opening in Oncology." She shakes her head as if she can't believe her luck. "I feel I can tell patients who come into Oncology, 'I've been there, I can help you through.' I see the calming effect that has."

Nancy says her lymphedema didn't appear until well after her treatments for breast cancer. "I was always one of the healthiest people I knew. Until I got breast cancer, I'd never had health problems. Then it seemed like everything happened. A year after I was done with the breast cancer treatments, I had carpal tunnel. It was in my right wrist, the same side as my breast cancer. I was lucky, I guess, because I didn't have lymphedema at the time, though I told the surgeon lymphedema might be a problem and he took some precautions.

"Then, my husband and I took a little vacation at a bed and breakfast in the country. The woman who ran the bed and breakfast had lymphedema. Every evening we'd see her in the family room of the house with her arm elevated on pillows and encased in a pump. She'd gone to a conference at Stanford and she knew tons about lymphedema. I learned a lot from her. She attributed her lymphedema to a flu shot she'd had in that arm—she said she just didn't think about it.

"After hearing her story, I was much more aware of the seriousness of lymphedema. Because of the type of nursing I'd done before, I'd never really seen women with it.

"My own lymphedema started nearly two years after I was finished with the cancer treatments." She slips her sweater off and bends both her arms in front of herself as if to show the comparison. Though there is no swelling in her hand, one arm is somewhat larger than the other.

Once lymphedema set in, Nancy says she tried to elevate her arm as much as possible, though she admits she was frustrated and scared that it would get out of control. "I was lucky I was in medicine, and because I met that woman on my trip. I had some idea what to do."

She started treatments by going in for lymphatic massage every other day for two or three weeks. During those treatments she didn't see much reduction in the swelling. "The physical therapist," she says, "wasn't very encouraged because of the amount of radiation I'd had. My goal was to maintain and not let it get any worse, though I think there's been a slight increase in the last year. If I dedicated the hour and a half to two hours a day to work with it, maybe it wouldn't be getting worse, I don't know. Anyway, the lymphatic massage treatment was one of the most pleasant, gentle, and relaxing things I have ever experienced."

Nancy says that even after lymphatic massage she continues to bandage at night and to do self-massage on her arm, particularly when she's noticed an episode of swelling. "At first, my husband helped with my back. We worked steadily on it for quite a while, though I still have a pocket of lymphedema there. When I didn't see improvement in my arm, I requested the pump." (We'll discuss the pump in a later chapter.)

"But the pump was not for me. It hurt and I had to dedicate so much time to it. I tried it for about a month, setting aside time every day for it. I realized it was beginning to seem like it was ruling my life—everything else I wanted to do, all the activities of life like school committees, programs for my children, gardening, didn't allow me time to sit and be on the pump. I decided I was not going to let it rule my life, so I gave up on it. I had one patient who used the pump, however, and had good results. She still tells me she is happy as a clam with it.

"After that, I started doing self-massage also and intermittently bandaging, but I still didn't see any change. It was hard, too; some nights I just wanted to go to bed and sleep with nothing on my arm.

"Now that I am in Radiation Oncology, I see patients with lymphedema and I refer them to physical therapy for treatments in lymphatic massage. And to those who don't have lymphedema, I talk about general precautions. It's another thing that makes me glad I know how to be of help."

Nancy says she also tried using the Reid sleeve, a type of wrap that is somewhat like the bandages but that straps onto the arm (or the leg in lower extremity lymphedema). "Because I see a lot of information coming across my desk, I found out about the sleeve, and the pictures made the Reid sleeve look tolerable. I wanted to just be able to slip my arm in the sleeve and go to bed at night. It took more than six months for my insurance company to agree to pay for it.

"But when I got the sleeve, I found out it's enormous, and not at all what I'd imagined. But, as cumbersome as it is, I do still use it at times."

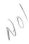

She holds out her arm again and fingers a silver chain bracelet on her wrist. "I use this as a sort of gauge," she says. "There are times when the bracelet's so tight around my wrist it settles into a position where it leaves big dents." Today, the bracelet swings loosely around her wrist as she twists it. "It helps me gauge the degree of swelling. When my arm is actively swelling, I'll bandage at night and wear a Juzo sleeve during the day. When it's not a problem, I use the Reid sleeve alone, though I've found that the bandaging is most effective. I have discovered a new Juzo sleeve that has silicon grippers at the top. It's a lot better than the old sleeves, because it stays up. I couldn't work with the older models, but I have no trouble at all with the new silicon one."

For a moment she does not speak, and sits tipping her head. Finally she says, "Do you know what really sort of bothers me? When I show someone my arm and they say, 'That's not so bad.'

I guess it isn't that bad from the perspective of somebody else, but to me it seems so big and obvious." She lightly rubs the edema around her elbow, then slips back into the sweater. "I have to shop differently now. I find myself wearing sweaters to cover my arm even in the summer. I dread that summer is coming because of the heat." She takes a big breath, lets out a sigh.

"I see women taking all kinds of measures to deal with their swelling, wearing gloves and sleeves and going regularly for treatments, and they aren't experiencing so much lymphedema as I have. Maybe if I had that kind of attitude, my arm wouldn't be as swollen—I don't know.

"I do take care, however. I don't ignore my arm and I don't jeopardize its condition, but I don't let it run my life, either. Our family's just like everyone else's, I guess, we're so busy. My son has tennis at seven o'clock, my daughter has to be at high school at seven forty-five. I have to be at work by eight." She laughs again; it is obvious she loves doing all she does. "Now, how am I going to be able to put more time into lymphedema?

"I guess the best thing that has come out of this last few years is my sense of living better each day. You know," she says, "in a way, that year dealing with cancer turned out to be one of the best years of my life. I spent time with myself, and my family, and with friends I normally never have time with. Even if I'd known ahead of time I'd get lymphedema, I would have chosen to go through everything I did for the cancer. I've had four years of health, and four good years with my family. That's not so bad, after all."

17

Compression with Vasopneumatic Pumps

THOUGH THEY ARE NOW BEING USED less frequently, vasopneumatic pumps have been used for over twenty-five years in the treatment of lymphedema. In fact, until the last decade or so, pumps and compression garments were the only treatments available. Though other, more effective, treatments have emerged, pumps are still being prescribed by some doctors and used by thousands of people with lymphedema.

The pump is an electric compression device. It consists of a small pump attached by plastic tubing to an inflatable sleeve that fits over your arm or leg. The machine pumps air into the sleeve, causing the bag to inflate, and then after a set number of seconds, it turns off, allowing the sleeve to deflate. The cycle of inflation and deflation goes on as long as the machine is on. The newer pumps are programmed to inflate the sleeve starting at the most distal (farthest) part from your shoulder, the fingers, and to gradually inflate each subsequent section moving up your arm toward the shoulder. The theory is to "milk" the lymph fluid out of the swollen extremity.

In the vast majority of cases, these pumps have little or no lasting beneficial effects.

Dr. Michael Foeldi, world-renowned in the field of lymphology, says that to squeeze fluid from an extremity with lymphedema toward an area that has had regional lymph node dissection "defies an understanding of basic anatomy and physiology."[1] In the lymphatic system, the arm and the trunk on that side of the body flow into the same axillary nodes (nodes that may have been damaged by radiotherapy or even removed). The pump's action of pushing fluid from the arm into the trunk simply increases the swelling in the trunk on that side. The pump does nothing to move the protein-rich lymph fluid into a different lymphatic quadrant that could drain the fluid away or break down the impurities.[2]

An analogy that may help explain this concept is of a swimming pool that has no drain. If you pump water in the pool from the deep end to the shallow end, it will eventually filter back to the deep end. To decrease the volume of water in the pool, the pump needs to drain *outside* the pool. It is the same with lymphedema. Without drainage, the fluid often quickly filters back to the arm when the person stops using the compression pump.

At the 1993 International Congress of Lymphology there was general agreement that a pump used by itself is not an effective treatment for lymphedema. If a pump is used at all, it should be used in conjunction with MLD® and a comprehensive treatment program. It should also be set at a low pressure.[3]

Problems can develop with ongoing use of a compression pump. It may cause a fibrosis, or thickening, to develop where the fluid accumulates and has a higher concentration at the top of the arm. The 1995 Consensus Document of the International Society of Lymphology suggests that care must be taken to prevent the patient from developing a fibrosclerotic ring on the arm where the inflatable sleeve ends.[4]

Additionally, the pump may damage remaining, healthy lymph vessels.[5] Patients may not have been given adequate training or sufficient information to use the machines in the most effective or safe manner. When the pumps are not effective in reducing the swelling, or if swelling returns immediately, a common response is to increase the pressure in the pump or to increase the time spent using it, both of which are contraindicated. The pressures used are often too great for the fragile lymphatic vessels and can damage them. At a minimum, the higher pressure compresses the lymphatic vessels and does not allow them to work.

Patients frequently report that home use of the pump works for a while and then gradually becomes less and less effective as fibrosis develops or as lymphatic pathways become damaged. As it becomes less effective, they get discouraged and eventually discontinue use of the pump. Any therapist who works a great deal with lymphedema will know of patients with a pump in the closet or for sale.

In conclusion, we would discourage people from using a pump. But if you do use a pump, please consider the following guidelines:

- Use a pump *only* under the supervision of a therapist trained in comprehensive lymphatic treatment.

- Use a pump with segmental gradient compression starting at your fingers and moving up toward the shoulder.

- Use the pump along with a comprehensive treatment program that includes lymphatic drainage, bandaging, and exercise.

- Keep the pressure low—never higher than 35 mm Hg.

- Practice self-massage to the neck and trunk before, during, and after pumping. It is very important to clear an area for the fluid to move to.

- Never use the pump if you have swelling in your trunk.

- Especially with primary lymphedema, be cautious, and watch the groin area closely for problems.

- Use extreme caution with primary lymphedema, as pumping can contribute to edema in the genital area.

- Never use the pump if you have an infection.

- Discontinue use of the pump if it causes pain.

- If your physician recommends a compression pump, ask

about other options for treatment. Share with your doctor any information you might have regarding complex decongestive therapy. Contact the National Lymphedema Network or check the Internet to obtain information that might further educate your physician.

In the next chapter you will find Carolyn's story. Carolyn experienced lymphedema after treatments for cancer, and, at that time, a pump was prescribed. She recounts her experience using the pump.

18

Carolyn: Using a Vasopneumatic Pump

CAROLYN WORKS AS A TEACHER'S AIDE at a grade school. She has an eager, alert expression. She is short, not much over five feet tall, with curly black hair. It is hard to imagine kids being able to put much over on her. She is in her early forties, rounded and attractive.

"I work in the learning support room with kids with learning disorders." She adds that she also tutors seven foreign students in English.

The T-shirt she wears is short-sleeved. One arm is noticeably, maybe three or four inches, larger than the other. She is wearing no jewelry on that arm. "It's the fourth year I've worked at the school," she says. "I subbed one year. The next year the person who was working with the disabled kids left her job, and I got it. Within a week at my new job I found out I had a recurrence of the cancer. It had gone to my bones, mostly to my pelvis." She points to a spot on top of her head. "There was a spot here on my head, too, and in six more places.

"Because I got such terrible hot flashes," she says, "I had quit the Tamoxifen the doctors prescribed. When the cancer came back I felt real bad, as if that's what caused it. But the doctor said the cancer would have come back anyway sometime."

She says she had chemo again and radiation the second time, and Taxol, which she had to discontinue because of the horrible pain it gave her. "I'm on Megase now. Four pills a day. The hot flashes aren't as bad, except every morning before I go to work I have some. But I still have water retention and weight gain. My appetite is really up.

"The cancer has disappeared everywhere but maybe the last spot in my pelvis."

She has spoken directly about her cancer. She speaks equally directly about her lymphedema, which developed right after her mastectomy. She asked the doctor about it, but he did not seem to have any idea what could be done. "It was the clerk at the place where I bought my prosthesis who told me about lymphedema," she says. "The store had pictures on the walls of people who had it really bad. Until then, I still didn't know where to get help.

"My mother bought me a Lymphopress pump. It cost her three thousand dollars. I used it for four years. Every day I would sit for two hours at night with my arm in the pump and it would take the swelling down. But a couple of hours later my arm would swell up again. Finally, three months ago, I was referred to a therapist. She taught me drainage massage and exercises and showed me how to bandage.

"She was surprised when I told her I had a pump. She asked what pressure I had it at and I told her eighty millimeters of pressure. She quickly advised me, 'Set it lower. It shouldn't be any more than thirty-five millimeters.' She was so emphatic that I set it lower even before I turned it on again.

"I have lymphedema mostly in my lower arm and a little in my upper arm." She holds out her arm. She turns it, inspects it. "It's going down now. But the therapist said it might have weighed fifteen pounds more than the other before I started treatment."

She circles her wrist with the fingers of her other hand; they come half an inch short of meeting. "It's really down," she says. "Before, I couldn't get my fingers within an inch and a half of coming together." She says she also has lymphedema in her trunk and chest, and in front of her armpit. She indicates where in her armpit the swelling was. "But that has gone away since I began treatment a couple of months ago.

"After all the trouble I've had in the last four years, I'm real good about massaging and bandaging every night. And I do the exercises and then rewrap before I go to bed. I love this regimen, because I don't have to spend hours on the machine anymore." Then she adds, "But a couple of times I've used the machine when it was hot and my arm was really swollen."

She adds she rarely eats anything with salt in it anymore. "And I really am careful to drink lots of water. Water really helps keep down the swelling in my arm. I really notice the difference when I don't drink it enough. In fact, last weekend I got some sort of bug and I had diarrhea. And I got dehydrated and my arms really swelled up. So, I'm convinced drinking water is real important for me.

"And I found something else that I think is really helping: I started going to an herbalist. She's teaching me that my body is a healing machine. She's teaching me to think positively and not to associate every little ache and pain with cancer. And I'm learning to tell the cancer to go away." She laughs, "I say, 'Cancer, you're not welcome here. You've got to go.'

"The herbalist has taught me to pretend I am on a cliff and if I make one misstep I'll fall down a thousand-foot drop. And I picture grabbing every crack, every hold I can, to keep going, just like I do to keep away the cancer."

19

Breathing Exercises

BEFORE WE GET INTO what might traditionally be considered exercise, we'll start with a particular kind of deep breathing called *belly breathing*, or breathing with the diaphragm. It is a form of exercise that is effective in moving fluid, and we will weave it throughout the exercise regimens.

Breathing is something we don't have a choice about, but *how* we breathe is something we can choose. Learning to breathe in a way that moves your abdominal muscles is an easy way to create a gentle continual pumping action to the central lymphatic vessel in the chest cavity, stimulating the flow of lymph. When you breathe in, using your abdominal muscles, the pressure in the chest cavity changes, because the belly breath moves your diaphragm. When you exhale, the pressure changes once again. This back-and-forth alternation in pressure acts like a pump on the large lymphatic trunk that runs up through the chest cavity and drains into the venous system at the neck.

Watch how babies breathe. They practice belly breathing naturally. When a baby breathes in, its belly puffs out like a balloon. When it breathes out, its belly flattens again.[1]

Here's how the anatomy of it works. The diaphragm is a large sheet of muscle located right underneath the lungs, separating the lung cavity from the abdominal cavity. When it is relaxed it looks like a dome. As you inhale, the diaphragm contracts and pulls downward. Its downward movement creates a negative pressure, and the lower lobes of the lungs fill with air. As your diaphragm moves downward, it pushes on the abdominal cavity and your belly expands outward to accommodate the extra air in your lungs. When you exhale, the diaphragm relaxes and lets go, returning to its dome position, forcing air out of the lungs and flattening the belly.[1]

When you breathe with the belly, or the diaphragm, in this way, your breath becomes deep and relaxed. This allows your lungs to fill with oxygen all the way to the bottom, and it promotes a pumping action in the lymph vessels of your chest cavity.

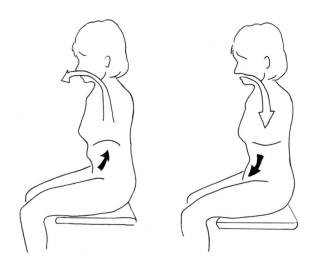

Figure 19-1. Abdominal breathing

Many people do not take advantage of the relaxation and increased oxygen that this abdominal breathing provides. Instead, they move only the upper parts of their chest, with raised shoulders, rather than allowing their lungs to fill fully with air. Many of us fall into shallow breathing patterns for a variety of reasons—stress responses, reaction to pain, respiratory problems, allergies, and that forever-present sense that we need to hold our stomach in. Many of us even hold our breath at times.

In order to promote a healthy environment for your body, you want to provide the most possible oxygen and cause a change in the chest cavity pressure, so your lymphatics will pump efficiently. A smooth, even, belly-breathing pattern is important.

Now, to actually practice the skill.

How to Breathe with Your Abdomen

First, concentrate on your breathing: become aware of how you actually breathe. As essential as breathing is, most of us are never aware of our breathing patterns. To concentrate on it for a moment, sit in a straight-backed chair with your feet flat on the floor. Rest your hands gently against your abdomen. Without trying to change or force any particular type of breathing, just notice whether your belly is expanding or flattening as you breathe. You might find it easier to close your eyes while you focus on your next few breaths.

If you noticed that your belly is expanding into your hands as you inhale, you are probably breathing with your diaphragm (at least in part). If your hands are still and your belly doesn't move much with breathing, you are most likely breathing from your upper chest.

The next step is to start to practice abdominal breathing.

Stay in the same upright position in the chair. Take in a deep breath through your nose and then exhale completely through your mouth, flattening your belly and squeezing out every last bit of air. Emptying the lungs completely and removing all the stale air from the bottom of the lungs automatically stimulates a diaphragmatic breath. Breathe in through your nose, and notice how your belly expands. Repeat the sequence again. Let the air out through your mouth, making sure your belly flattens. Try another one or two breaths this way. If you get light-headed, try to slow down your inhalation, and pause before breathing in again.

After the first couple of breaths, continue a gentle breathing pattern, inhaling through your nose and exhaling through your mouth, allowing your tummy to gently expand and contract. It is not necessary to breathe with a giant breath—just one that goes to the bottom of your lungs, while your chest remains still. It may help to keep your hands on your belly and try to gently push your abdomen into your hands as you breathe in.

If using an image helps, picture a balloon in your lower stomach that inflates when you inhale and deflates when you breathe out.

Some Tips

- Start practicing with only four or five breaths, and slowly increase your practice time to one minute or longer. Practice several times a day.

- In the beginning, you might find it helpful to practice abdominal breathing while lying down on your bed or on the floor. Bend your knees and place your feet comfortably apart.

- If you feel light-headed, dizzy, or anxious, you may be breathing too deeply or too quickly. If this happens, stop practicing for a moment and breathe normally until the symptoms pass.

- Be patient. At first this way of breathing may seem awkward; some people wonder how this could possibly be the correct method of breathing. [2]

As you practice and generally become more aware of your breathing, this belly-breathing pattern becomes more natural, and you may find yourself automatically doing it throughout your day. It is a simple and effective way to stimulate the lymphatic system all day long.

20

How to Exercise with Lymphedema

WE TAKE IT FOR GRANTED that exercise is good for us. But do we do it? Probably not. We might take a stab at it now and then, maybe join a health club, or make a pact with our best friend. But honestly, how many of us follow through? How many stick with it? Probably not too many.

If ever there was a time to find an exercise program and keep at it, that time is now. When it comes to breast cancer, one study showed that women who exercise four hours a week have 37 percent less incidence of breast cancer than sedentary women.[1] These studies also suggest that exercise can be helpful in decreasing the risk of recurrence.

Women who exercise regularly generally have a lower percentage of body fat. Body fat generates more estrogen in the system, and puts us at higher risk for breast cancer. Obesity, it turns out, also puts us at higher risk for developing lymphedema.[2]

Though numerous studies cite the positive effects of exercise on breast cancer, there are none yet that indicate what part exercise plays in reducing lymphedema. It is unfortunate, but lymphedema in general has not been studied much. But although there is no study or trial to guide them, practitioners know exercise works.[3] Therefore, all therapy and rehabilitation programs for lymphedema incorporate exercise into their decongestive lymphatic therapy.[4]

Before you begin an exercise program, though, a word of

warning. Some exercises, particularly if they are not carried out with moderation and persistence, can actually be harmful. I remember one woman I saw as a patient. She had been protecting her arm for two years in fear of developing lymphedema when she was advised by her surgeon to go out and exercise it actively. In following her doctor's orders, she did, indeed, develop lymphedema, which has never completely gone away, even with treatment.

Exercise to treat lymphedema comes in several different types, four of which we'll cover here. Each type has a different treatment goal.

1. Lymph drainage exercises. These are simple mobility exercises performed in a specific sequence that pumps the fluid through the lymphatic pathways. They help to drain lymph away from congested areas and into areas of improved drainage.

2. Stretching and flexibility exercises. These exercises help achieve mobility, the ability to move muscles and joints through their full range of motion. *Flexibility* refers to the degree of normal motion, while *stretching* refers to the process of elongating muscles and other soft tissues.[5] After breast cancer surgery, women may have tightness in the pectoral area on the chest or decreased shoulder mobility. This may interfere with normal lymph or venous drainage from the arm.[6]

3. Strengthening. This refers to building the power of the muscle to improve endurance and capability of performance. The stronger the muscle, the better able it is to perform without overexertion or fatigue. It has been reported that progressive resistive training can increase lymphatic flow.[6]

4. Aerobic exercise. Dr. Kenneth Cooper defines this as "exercise which demands large quantities of oxygen for prolonged periods to force the body to improve those systems responsible for transportation of oxygen."[7] More simply, this means sustained exercise for fifteen to twenty minutes using your large muscles.

Goals of Exercise

The reasons for exercising are varied. The primary goals of exercising to treat lymphedema are to move lymph fluid and to reduce swelling. More specifically, exercise should:

- Pump the muscles to move lymph from the congested areas into an area where it can more easily drain. The first emphasis is to clear the trunk of your body. Only after your trunk is cleared do you exercise to drain your arm.

- Increase mobility of the shoulder girdle and spine. In the chapter entitled "Breast Cancer" in the book *Physical Therapy for the Cancer Patient*, the author reports that a common problem after breast cancer is decreased mobility and strength of the involved arm, particularly the shoulder girdle (which involves the shoulder blade, collarbone, shoulder, and upper arm).[8]

- Increase muscle strength and tone. Decreased strength can occur in the arm after breast cancer. Most often, diminution in strength is caused by disuse, pain, imbalances in posture, or fear of using the arm. Loss of strength can happen rapidly. Strengthening may allow you to do more activity without triggering the lymphatic response with increased fluid. If you have had a mastectomy, the muscles of the shoulder girdle and shoulder blade may weaken if you unconsciously guard the area and do not move your muscles naturally. Or the development of scar tissue can make your shoulder pull toward the front of the trunk. This can result in improper posture. It is important to overcome these tendencies and to restore muscle balance to the upper trunk.

- Improve circulation. One method of improving lymph flow is to pump the blood vessel. This pumping can stimulate a stretch reflex in the lymph vessel, causing it to contract and move lymph fluid.

- Improve body awareness, and promote a sense of general well-being. Regular aerobic exercise can cause the body to secrete hormones called endorphins. Endorphins have been shown to be associated with feelings of euphoria and well-being. Endorphins are also powerful analgesics. It is believed that endorphins can be released even with exercise of relatively mild intensity.[9]

If you have a set of bandages or a compression garment, wear either of them during exercise. Bandages, particularly, increase pressure against the skin during the exercise workout. This pressure, coupled with the contraction of your muscles, encourages the lymph to move. A support garment can be worn during exercise as well, but its specific purpose is to *maintain* the reduction of swelling, not necessarily to reduce it.

Some of you may not have access to complete decongestive therapy and/or bandages. If so, the exercises can still be carried out with some benefit to lymph flow.[10] Learning to breathe using your diaphragm and belly will stimulate lymph circulation in your trunk. Your muscles can still act as a pump against the lymph vessels, and your circulatory system will be pumping as well. Exercising without bandages or garments is better than not exercising at all. A note of caution: Do not substitute Ace wraps for the short-stretch bandages. They are not intended for use in reducing lymphedema, as they do not provide enough pressure to move lymph. They may even cause interruption in lymph flow. (See chapter 14, "Compression Using Bandages.")

As for how much exercising to do and how fast to do it, use your arm as a monitor. If it swells, cut back some and build up more slowly. The program we suggest is not a recipe that fits everyone. No program does. In order to get the most benefit, you'll need to tweak and modify it to meet your own individual needs.

For example, if you had a previous back problem or shoulder

problem for which you were already doing exercises, you'll need to consider that in your regimen. There may be any number of factors that do not allow you to carry out all the exercises suggested in this text. Please get the input or advice of a trained therapist before you begin. The exercises we highlight should be taken as examples of a program you may want to consider. They are not all-inclusive, nor are they, by any means, the only effective exercises. Many routines can prove successful.

Again, use common sense. If you overdo, your arm may swell a bit more, but don't worry—you will probably be able to quickly reduce the swelling. If you have had an active day with lots of physical activity, let up on your exercises a bit. If you are feeling fatigued or tired before exercising one day, don't press; take that into account and adjust your program. Your program should not be rigid, but flexible and persistent.

Principles of Exercise

Here is a recap of the guiding principles to keep in mind as you are designing your program:

* Use some form of compression on your arm if it's available, especially as you begin your exercise program.

* Start very slowly with few repetitions and wait until the next day to see how your arm has responded.

* Gradually increase the repetitions, always using your arm as a guide to how much you can do.

* Make sure to continue a smooth breathing pattern throughout the exercise routine. Overcome the tendency to hold your breath. Relax your abdominal muscles and practice breathing into your belly.

* Use proper posture to open up all channels of possible fluid movement. Good posture also facilitates a good breathing pattern. What I mean by good posture is that the feet should be well planted, making a stable base, with the

knees unlocked, tucking your buttocks, keeping your chest up, shoulders relaxed and dropped down, head back and squarely over the shoulders.

◆ Always move slowly and deliberately, being aware of what muscles you are using. Concentrate on the movement. Pause between repetitions.

◆ *Never* cause pain. The old adage "No pain, no gain" is not accurate. You should never experience any significant discomfort while you exercise (other than the discomfort and bulk of all those bandages).

When You Should *Not* Exercise:

◆ When you are ill with a fever.

◆ If you experience chest pain.

◆ If you experience sudden shortness of breath or unusual fatigue.

◆ When you have recurring leg pain or cramps.

◆ If you experience an acute onset of nausea during exercise.

◆ If you feel disoriented or confused.

◆ When you have had recent bone, back, or neck pain that is not relieved with rest.

◆ If you have an irregular heartbeat.[11]

◆ ◆ ◆

Now, to the actual exercises—but be sure to consult with your doctor before starting your exercise program, or during it if you experience any problems.

21

Special Exercises for People with Lymphedema

IN THIS CHAPTER we will present some examples of exercise programs for each category outlined in the previous chapter: lymph drainage exercises, stretching exercises, strengthening exercises, and aerobic exercises. While it is best to follow a comprehensive exercise program, the first and most important exercises for those with lymphedema are the lymph drainage exercises.

Lymph Drainage Exercises

These exercises should always start with four to five abdominal breaths, with a contraction just strong enough so you can feel it. Don't force the breathing; you do not need to have the largest possible contraction.

1. **Pelvic Tilt.** Lie on your back with your knees bent and feet flat. Pull up and in with the abdominal muscles, flattening your lower back into the bed or to the floor.

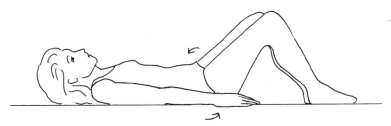

Figure 21-1. Pelvic tilt

2. **Partial Sit-up with Breathing.** Get in the same position as in #1. Breathe into your belly. As you exhale, lift up your head and shoulders.

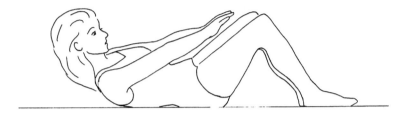

Figure 21-2. Partial sit-up with breathing

3. **Neck Rotation.** Turn your head slowly to the right to the count of five as you breathe in. Return to the center as you exhale. Repeat to the left.

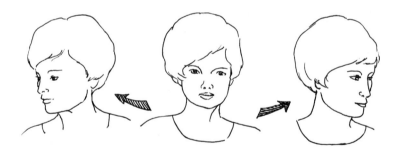

Figure 21-3. Neck rotation

4. **Head Tilt.** Tilt your head to the right, allowing your ear to drop toward your shoulder. Maintain this position for five seconds, then slowly bring your head back to the center. Repeat to the other side.

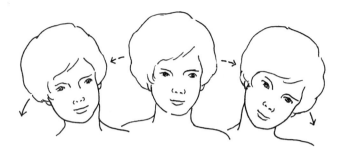

Figure 21-4. Head tilt

5. **Shoulder Shrug.** Shrug both shoulders, lifting them toward your ears as you breathe in. Then return to a relaxed position. Next, pull your shoulders down as far as possible, then return to the relaxed position.

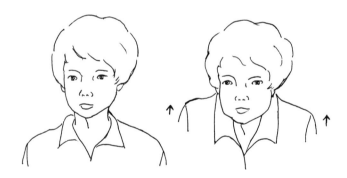

Figure 21-5. Shoulder shrug

6. **Shoulder Roll.** Lift the shoulders up toward the ears, then rotate the shoulders back and then drop them down, making a smooth, continuous, circular motion.

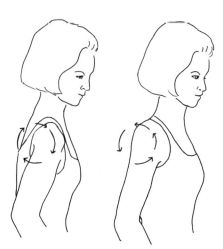

Figure 21-6. Shoulder roll

7. **Shoulder Blade Squeeze.** Bend your elbows to a right angle. Now, keep your elbows close to your body, and pull them toward the center of your back, squeezing the shoulders blades together.

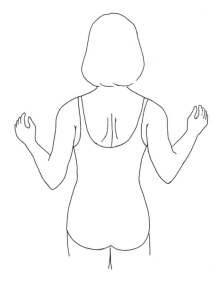

Figure 21-7. Shoulder blade squeeze

8. **Isometric Hand Press.** Place the palms of your hands together, with your elbows bent and arms at shoulder level. Push your palms together firmly, breathing in to the count of four, then relaxing and breathing out to the count of four.

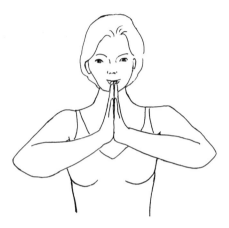

Figure 21-8. Isometric press

9. **Shoulder Rotation.** With the arms at shoulder height, rotate the palms outward slowly, so the palms are facing upward. Then rotate the arms inward.

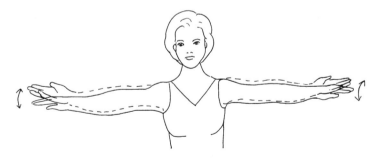

Figure 21-9. Shoulder rotation

10. **Elbow Bend.** Sit with your arm extended on a table or counter at shoulder height. Bend your elbow, pulling your

fingers toward your shoulder. Come up as far as you are able with the bandages on your arm. Return to the start position.

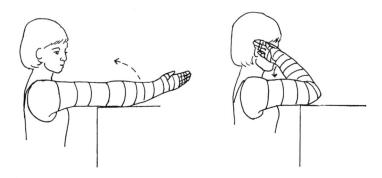

Figure 21-10. Elbow bend

11. **Wrist Circle.** Rotate your fist in small circles, isolating the movement to the wrist only. Rotate first in one direction, then the other.

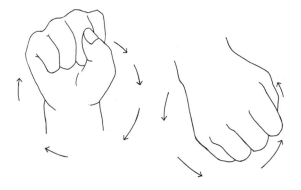

Figure 21-11. Wrist circle

12. **Fist Clench.** Open your hands and stretch your fingers, spreading them apart. Then slowly clench each hand to make a fist. Hold for three seconds, then relax.

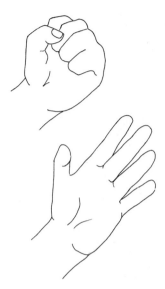

Figure 21-12. Fist clench

13. **Finger Exercise.** Hold your hands in front of you with the palms together. Separate matching pairs of fingers away from each other, one pair at a time, then reverse the sequence. As an additional exercise, press your fingers side to side, keeping them together.

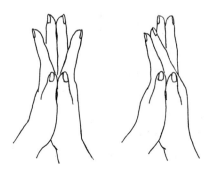

Figure 21-13. Finger exercise

14. **Breathing.** Practice belly breathing again.

After you complete these lymph drainage exercises, it is a good idea to lie down and relax for a few minutes (or longer), with your arm supported and elevated on a pillow.

Stretching and Flexibility Exercises

We recommend stretching just short of the point at which your muscle or joint will feel pain, then maintaining that position for several seconds. Stretching should be done slowly and with deliberation, from a well-aligned position, taking care that you keep up a smooth, even breathing pattern throughout.

As mentioned earlier, lack of flexibility in the shoulder girdle and trunk after breast cancer can be due to tightness of the scar tissue or connective tissue. This tissue responds best to low-force, long-duration stretching.[1] Tightness can also be caused by your holding your arm in a protected position and not moving it freely. If your arm is immobilized, it can quickly stiffen up, which can contribute to additional problems.

There are hundreds of other stretching and flexibility programs besides those we will mention here. Many excellent books give good information on stretching. Two strong books that seem very user-friendly are *Sport Stretch* by Michael Alter[1] and *Essential Guide to Stretching* by Chrissie Gallagher-Mundy.[2] Though the emphasis in our examples is mostly on the health of your shoulder and shoulder girdle, you cannot help but benefit if you incorporate an entire body stretching program, such as these books recommend, into your routine. Modify your program as you need, but remember, never force yourself or cause yourself unnecessary pain.

Stretches for the Shoulder

1. **Cane Exercise.** Use a broomstick or cane. Hold the stick on the top of your chest and below your chin with an undergrip (palms facing toward ceiling). Lift the stick up over your head to the back of your shoulders. If you can't lift the stick over your head, lift it as high as you can. Hold this position for three seconds, then return to the start position.

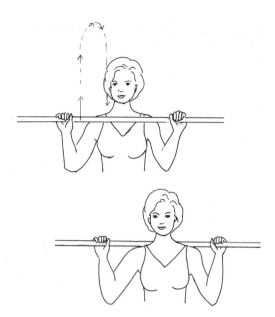

Figure 21-14. Cane exercise

2. **Door or Corner Stretch.** Stand facing a corner or open doorway. Raise your elbows, keeping them below your shoulders, and rest them against the wall. Lean your entire body forward. Maintain this stretch for fifteen to twenty seconds. You can vary this exercise and stretch different parts of the chest by gradually raising your arms higher.

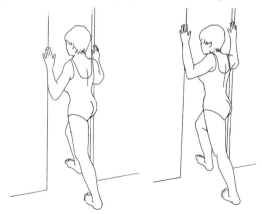

Figure 21-15. Door or corner stretch

3. **Towel Stretch.** Hold each end of a towel behind your back, with one arm behind your lower back and the other arm overhead. Pull the towel up and down as if your were drying your back.

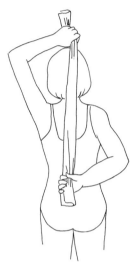

Figure 21-16. Towel stretch

4. **Hands and Knees Stretch.** Rest on your hands and knees with your arms slightly in front of your shoulders. Rock back toward your heels, stretching your shoulders.

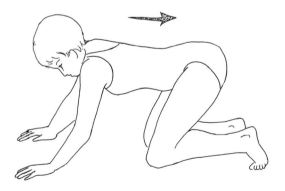

Figure 21-17. Hands and knees stretch

Strengthening: Progressive Exercises Adding Resistance

Gradually you can add other exercises that include some resistance. One method of giving your workout resistance is to use a Theraband (a stretchy elastic band color-coded for different levels of resistance that can be cut into varying lengths). A Theraband increases the workload, helping to build muscle tone and strength.

If you do add a Theraband or some other form of resistance to your workout, start slowly. Begin with a low resistance and few repetitions, and gradually increase over several months, especially if you have not previously been physically active or exercising regularly.

If you want to use weights, start with one to two pounds, gradually increasing your repetitions and the weight. Always monitor your arm for increased swelling. If swelling persists for more than twenty-four hours after a workout, you need to decrease the number of repetitions or the amount of weight you're using.[3]

There are several areas to focus on when strengthening. The first is the shoulder and shoulder girdle. I find that many women have lost strength in their upper back and around their shoulder blade. Second, all the muscle groups of the arm can benefit from strengthening to build up the arm so it will not be overloaded or fatigued by the activities of daily living. It is also beneficial to work the arm muscles with light resistance, because this pumps the muscles assisting with lymph drainage. Especially important are those in the path of alternative lymphatic drainage, such as the deltoid, which lies over the top of the shoulder, or the triceps, which is in the back of the upper arm. The third basic area that *all* people need to strengthen is the abdominal muscles. Remember to avoid contracting the abdominal muscles continually for long periods of time, as this does not allow you to belly breathe.

It would be overwhelming to cover all the exercises you might be able to do. Since each exercise program for lymphedema needs to be individualized, it would be valuable for you to seek the advice of a trained therapist to evaluate your specific needs and to help establish a program designed to meet your needs. Following are a few examples of exercises we have used with our patients.

Using Theraband or Rubber Tubing

1. **Lawn Mower Pull.** Stand on one end of the Theraband and wrap the other end around your hand on the involved side. Bend over slightly, perhaps holding on to a counter or table. Pull your arm back as if you were starting a power lawn mower. Repeat five to seven times.

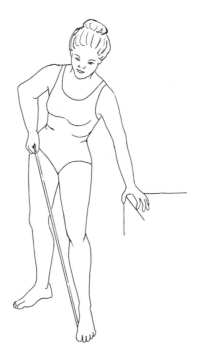

Figure 21-18. Theraband lawn mower pull

2. **Chest Pull.** Hold each end of the band at chest height. Pull out to the side, extending your arms out to the side while squeezing your shoulder blades together. Repeat five to seven times.

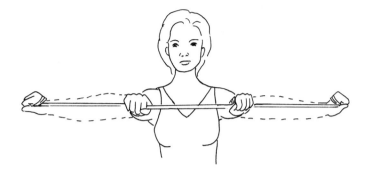

Figure 21-19. Theraband chest pull

Using Low Weight

Start these exercises with one-pound weights and build up to a maximum of three pounds.

1. **Arms out to Side.** Standing with a small weight in each hand, bring your arms out to the side and up to shoulder height. Hold this position for five seconds, then slowly lower your arms. Repeat five to seven times.

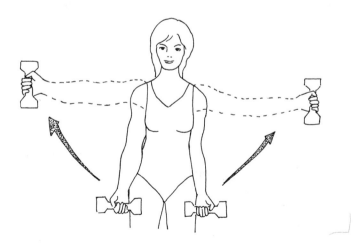

Figure 21-20. Arms out to side

2. **Reaching to the Ceiling.** Lie on your back. Holding the weight in the hand of your involved arm, point the extended arm toward the ceiling. Let your elbow bend down and then extend it up toward the ceiling again. Repeat five to seven times.

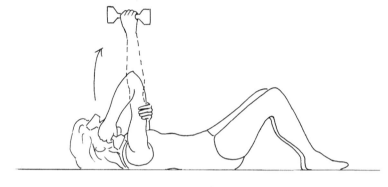

Figure 21-21. Reaching to the ceiling

Ethyfoam Roller Exercises

Other exercises may be added as needed or suggested by your therapist. Some exercises I have found useful include work with an ethyfoam roller four to six inches in diameter. This is a firm, Styrofoam-like roll. You lie on your back with the roll under your spine and do some breathing, balancing, arm movements, opposing movements with the arm and leg, and some rolling from side to side. This type of exercise has proven effective in orthopedic situations. I think it may also help to mobilize the spine and muscles along the side of the spine. Theoretically, this can influence the collateral lymph vessels, which carry the fluid across the watersheds to the normal quadrant. It also helps to mobilize the ribs, assists with improved breathing patterns, and promotes improved posture.

A physical therapist we know occasionally has patients purchase a "noodle," a 6-foot-long Styrofoam roll that is used in the summertime as a swimming pool floatation device. It is only about 3" wide and is softer material, but can be used if you cannot find an ethyfoam roller.

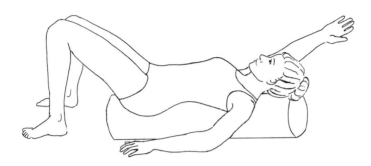

Figure 21-22. Ethyfoam roller

Gwen relates an experience with one of her first patients with lymphedema: She came in the week before I was scheduled to go to my first training program in lymphedema treatment. I didn't know about lymphatic massage or any other treatment techniques for lymphedema, but I did know about neck and back dysfunctions and was familiar with muscle spasms.

I plunged into treatment of her musculoskeletal dysfunctions and put her on one of these ethyfoam rollers. After working with the roller for several minutes, teaching her some diaphragm breathing, and giving her some postural pointers, we looked at her arm and were shocked to see that it had visibly decreased in size.

What I know now is that we cleared out her trunk to create room for the fluid to drain into. Her tight muscles along her spine, her stiff and rounded upper back, and her poor breathing patterns were contributing to some blockage of lymph flow, and working on these helped immediately. I have been using the roller ever since with lymphedema patients.

Therapy Ball or Gymnastic Ball

Another exercise tool is a called a therapy ball or gymnastic ball. These are large, strong balls that come in different sizes and are fun and versatile tools that can be used for a variety of exercises. You can sit on them, lie on your back to stretch over them, or lie over them on your stomach. The ball can also be used for different stretching, strengthening, and stabilization programs. Both the ball and the ethyfoam roller can be used at home on a regular basis. They can be purchased through a medical supply company or your health care provider's local physical therapy department. The large balls available in toy stores are often not strong enough for these exercises and should not be used. As always, consult with a therapist to help you find the most appropriate—and safe—exercises for your situation.

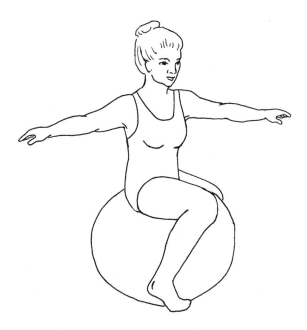

Figure 21-23. Therapy ball

Other Exercises

There is a wide variety of exercises that can benefit you if you have lymphedema. In chapter 7, "What Can I Do to Prevent Lymphedema?" we mentioned a video you might want to try that is available from the National Lymphedema Network. Many patients have found it helpful to practice Tai Chi or Qigong. Both provide slow, deliberate movements that focus on breathing and alignment. In chapter 26, Feather's story illustrates how Qigong has helped her.

Yoga, too, can be a wonderful help, with its focus on breathing, posture, tuning in to your body, and being with the movement. Belly dancing, tap dancing, ballet—anything that gets you moving and keeps you moving—can help as well.

When you pursue any kind of exercise, we recommend that you wear bandages or a support garment and follow the general guideline of using your arm as a monitor of how much you can do. With any exercise, it is important *not to overdo!* Start slowly, and gradually progress by increasing resistance and/or repetitions as you become more relaxed and accustomed to the exercise.

Overexercising, even with the gentle forms of Qigong, Tai Chi, and yoga, can cause an increase of fluid in the area, which is just what you're striving to avoid.

Aerobic Exercises

Aerobic exercise can serve you in many ways. The movement of the exercise coupled with the deep breathing it requires can cause a reduction in swelling by increasing lymph flow and improving the fluid balance in your body.[3] In addition, as your cardiovascular system works harder to pump the blood vessels during aerobic exercise, it stimulates the lymph vessels running next to the blood vessels. This also enhances lymph flow.

I usually suggest that women start an aerobic program with walking or bicycling. But a word of caution: Be careful not to do your exercise in the heat of the day. Exercise when it's cool, in the morning or in the evening. Or, if you are using a machine indoors, exercise in a cool, air-conditioned place. Be careful not to choose an activity that strains you or jars you, or one in which you could injure yourself.

Swimming and exercises in a pool are also excellent regimens. The pressure of the water helps to provide hydrostatic pressure to the arm and minimize swelling. Dr. Casley-Smith suggests scuba diving.[4] Some people use their old support garments while in the water for even better results. Water also helps to loosen up your shoulder girdle. Check with the local recreation centers or pools in your community to see what type of pool programs are available.

Aerobic exercise is also a realistic way to help lose weight and keep it off. Obesity has been suggested as a contributing factor in developing lymphedema.[5] Regular exercise can be an effective part of a weight-loss program.

With aerobics, it is recommended that you work toward a goal of twenty to thirty minutes of exercise (walking, jogging, dancing, etc.) four times a week.[6] In the course of our therapy, we have everyone who is medically able begin an aerobic exercise program. We progress very slowly over the course of treatment, which may take up to four weeks or longer. If you have not been exercising previously, start with five minutes and gradually increase over several weeks or months. Again, use your arm as a measure of how much you can do.

As you exercise, take your pulse at your wrist or neck while at rest and at different times during the workout. Make it your target to attain and maintain 60 percent of your maximum heart rate (this is 220 minus your age times 60 percent). The American College of Sports Medicine recommends you "accumulate 30 minutes or more of moderate intensity physical activity over the course of most days of the week."[7]

Though a lot of aerobic exercise requires no more equipment than a good pair of sports shoes, there is one apparatus that is especially good for upper-body movement. It is called a UBE, or upper-body exerciser. It is like a stationary bike for your arms. Our facility has a UBE, as do some health clubs and gyms.

We often recommend that our patients use the UBE. After wrapping the arm in bandages, we start the patient with one to two minutes on the machine, set to zero resistance. If your gym has a UBE, you can do the same thing. Warm up to it, though, and wear your bandages. Remember, it is better to err on the side

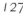

of less (and be cautious of trainers at the clubs, who may not be at all familiar with lymphedema and may be overzealous).

❖ ❖ ❖

You now have some idea of what you can do to take care of your lymphedema. No more procrastinating. No more unfulfilled promises. Start today. Find a friend to exercise with, pick an activity that you'd both enjoy, start slowly and with a small amount, and gradually increase. Set yourself up to be successful. After six months, you will see real benefits. We do in our clinic. Previous patients often stop by to visit, even years after treatment. They tell us the single greatest factor in successfully keeping their lymphedema under control has been sticking with a regular exercise program.

In the next chapter, Anita highlights the results her complete program has produced. She follows a commonsense regimen that incorporates some ideas of her own. You may want to consider it when designing yours.

22

Anita: A Committed Focus Yields Results

ABOUT A YEAR AFTER Anita and her husband moved to the area where they live now, her breast cancer was diagnosed. That was a little over two years ago.

Anita had been a nurse for twenty-five years, working in Oncology for the last sixteen. "I learned that the view of cancer from a patient's perspective is a lot different from that of a nurse's," she says. She has a warm way of speaking and a soft demeanor, indications she would be comforting as a nurse. "For sixteen years I had administered the same drugs I knew I'd be taking for my own cancer." Her voice softens. "It was amazing to be on the other side. It's so predictable when you're on the medical end of it: you do surgery, then chemotherapy, and, if the cancer comes back, maybe more treatment, then hospice, and…" her voice trails off. "I soon realized that wasn't the progression I intended for myself. I'll admit it was a very difficult time for me.

"As a nurse, I knew what worked and what didn't work. I knew the risks, including the risk of lymphedema. But, in a way, knowing is not really much help. Until you go through it, you don't know how it will feel to *you*."

Her arm and hand are covered with a compression sleeve. Her arm is slim, appearing no different in shape from her other one. She says that, after the diagnosis, she had a mastectomy and four sessions of chemotherapy, but she did not have radiation treatments.

"During treatment, I had two goals: to get rid of the cancer, and to guard against lymphedema. I talked with my surgeon about lymphedema, and he said that if swelling didn't develop right after surgery, it wasn't really considered lymphedema. I did have swelling in my chest after surgery due to bleeding, but with healing it went away.

"I went to work on a plan to restore my health. I wanted to get my arm mobility back and I wanted to expedite healing, so I started gentle exercising." She had always been pretty active, but she enrolled in a beginners' aerobics class while she was still in chemotherapy. "I could manage it about half the time, when I wasn't too washed out or sick from the chemo." All through chemo she had no changes in her arm, but she knew enough not to allow treatment to be given there. It was on vacation, nine months after treatment, that she had a sudden swelling in the arm. She and her husband had made a four-hour flight to Chicago to visit relatives. "I didn't know any precautions to take while flying." The day after they arrived, her lower arm and her hand swelled.

"I was out of town, away from home, and I really got worried, wondering if I should call my doctor, if I should go home, stay, or what. I thought if I could get home and get back to exercising and swimming, I might be able to help it. It was really frightening.

"Anyway, I decided to ride out the week of vacation and try a couple things I thought might help. The muscle in my lower arm was sore, so I tried putting heat on it. I know now that wasn't the thing to do. And I tried raising my arm on a pillow. The swelling didn't go away, but it didn't seem to get any worse either. When I got back home to my usual regimen, most of the swelling disappeared, but there was still a fullness in my upper arm."

She explains that her desire to limit problems before they get to be huge motivates her to stick to this treatment plan, though it is challenging. "I didn't realize at first that I would need to wrap my arm both day and night. I began to think about how to make this work. I struggled with my appearance, how the wrapping made me look like I'd had a major accident. It attracted immediate attention. I finally learned to tell people who asked, that the bandages were for protection." She laughs out loud. "It's funny, but nobody ever asked me what *kind* of protection. I don't know what I would have said if they had."

She says wrapping presented a real dilemma when it came to fitting into her clothes. "The bandages were so bulky, getting a long sleeve over them was impossible. I was wondering if I'd have to grapple with bandages for the rest of my life." Now she is able to wear a compression sleeve during the day, though she still wraps the arm in bandages most nights. "Before I got the sleeve, I found at first that the bandages would begin to itch and feel tight after about three or four hours, and I would look for things to distract myself with. The main distraction was eating. Then I started gaining weight and decided I was going to have a real problem if I didn't watch out." She finds that the compression sleeve allows a lot more freedom of movement and fits under clothes, and, she says, "I forget that it's there." She says she measures her arm regularly so she can determine what causes the swelling to flare up. "I'm getting a little sense of what I can and can't do."

Besides wrapping and wearing the sleeve, Anita is careful to use lotions that help maintain the health of her skin, and she is faithful to an exercise regimen. Her regimen started just a few weeks after her surgery, when her husband put up a basketball hoop and they began shooting hoops together. "It seemed like a logical thing for arm exercise, though I have to admit, winter put a crimp in it." She says that now she goes to a low-impact aerobics/dance class and yoga several times a week. "I've been incorporating lymphedema exercises into the yoga routines. It took me almost a year not to be sore after the yoga sessions, because I have some arthritis."

She admits her complete regimen takes a lot of effort. "When I realized it was going to take such a chunk of time, an hour and a half or so every day, to massage and exercise and bandage, I first tried to just squeeze it in without changing anything in my daily schedule. It didn't work. I had to allow time for it, to make it a real commitment. Sometimes I get discouraged when I consider I'm going to have to do some version of this for the rest of my life. It's like one more cost to having had breast cancer. But you can't let yourself lapse into self-defeating behaviors. Keeping my arm from ballooning is still important to me. I have the tools to deal with my lymphedema. I didn't have those before."

Part Three

◆

Beyond Conventional Treatments

23

Emotions and Lymphedema

THE EMOTIONAL DISCOMFORT of lymphedema can be as powerful as the physical. For some of us, this effect is the worst. The prospect of living with lymphedema can be scary, sad, and more than a little maddening.

Dr. Chandler, in his medical oncology practice, says the majority of his patients who encounter lymphedema become quite upset. "Fear, the heaviness of their arm, the feeling that nothing can be done, all cause a great deal of apprehension. Many women panic, or they just make themselves put up with it, or they live hiding it until somebody tells them how to get help. Some of my elderly women patients have had lymphedema for years and do not know that there is help available to them now."

With the exception of a few enlightened doctors, the medical community still tends to downplay or ignore the emotional component of lymphedema. However, psychologists and therapists have been counseling patients with the problem for decades. Three therapists, Ruth Bach, M. Ed., L.P.C., Izetta Smith, M.A., and Vicki Romm, L.C.S.W., generously share their experience and insight in this chapter.

Ruth Bach has been a counseling therapist for more than twenty years. She now heads the cancer counseling center at a large medical facility. She gives us the benefit of her experience not only as a therapist but also, in the next chapter, as a patient.

"Having lymphedema can be real depressing," Ruth says. "And for so many years, women were told they just had to live with their lymphedema. They often became depressed, and then they found no help for their depression."

A scientific study conducted in London between June 1990 and January 1991 illustrates Ruth's point.[1] One hundred women participated in the study. Half of them had breast cancer–related arm swelling, the other half did not. The women with swelling had experienced it for an average of about fifty months. All the participants were assessed as to both functional and psychiatric ability or impairment.

The study said that "Patients with arm swelling…experienced functional impairment, psychosocial maladjustment, and increased psychological morbidity." Those women also experienced difficulty in their home environments and in relationships within their families. The women who had no arm swelling appeared better able to assimilate the whole experience of breast cancer and to put it behind them and get on with their lives.

Ruth says, "In the past, it was like pulling teeth to get doctors to advise women to see a psychologist. And when they did, they felt such relief.

"A huge part of our job as counselors is to allow women to realize it is normal to feel the way they do. A woman feels validation when a counselor acknowledges to her that it is okay to pay attention to what she is feeling.

"We can also provide women with the knowledge that they are not alone, that they are not weird, that they or their bodies have not done something wrong to cause the cancer or the lymphedema. And we show them there are solutions, even if they have to search to find those solutions. Then, when many of the women see the results of physical therapy, they are thrilled. Most of them keep up with the program, wrapping and doing exercises."

Ruth adds that no matter how successful treatment is, no matter how much women might come to mental peace, there still may be misgivings. "When women realize this is ongoing and that they will be dealing with it the rest of their lives, they are likely to have regrets. It's all right not to like that this happened to you, but there is hope you can at least gain some control over it and can feel normal again. Counseling can have a huge effect in learning how to get through all of what we need to get through."

❖ ❖ ❖

Izetta Smith has counseled women with breast cancer and lymphedema for four years. She is articulate and emphatic about the effects of the diagnosis of cancer and treatment on the emotions of the women experiencing them.

"When women experience breast cancer," she says, "a range of different things can affect their day-to-day lives. There are those lucky women who don't experience many physical changes. But others undergo some real and immediate changes. Some women have almost instant menopause or perimenopause, with lowered libidos, hot flashes, and mood swings because of the changes in estrogen. There are also changes in their bodies after surgery. There is the need to deal with hair loss after chemotherapy. Normally, when we see a woman who is flooded with these day-to-day dealings, it's all she can talk about, all she can think about."

Izetta goes on to say that most women do handle these issues related to their cancer and manage to get on with living. "But," she says, "if a woman gets lymphedema a year or two after cancer, she finds another load to handle. With some women, it's almost as if this new problem stimulates the feelings of the original diagnosis of cancer, recycling the grief that came with the cancer. It can be a real, deep letdown."

She continues, "There are so many feelings of loss with cancer; big losses as well as little ones, some you may not feel for many years after the cancer. Cancer can truly bring a loss of innocence.

"Lymphedema can seem like another doorway into looking at what you have lost. In groups, women often say they feel lymphedema is a deformity. They find they can't button their sleeves, they have to quit wearing their jewelry, they have to wear different clothes. And, for some women, there is physical discomfort with lymphedema as well. Even if a woman does not have issues about her body image, even if the swelling is not important to her, she may have to deal with pain."

Vicki has been a practicing therapist for fifteen years. "I agree with Izetta," she says. "As women go along, they pass through the stages of treatment and healing and they begin to think they're done, and normally they come to a place of being okay with the breast cancer. Then the lymphedema is dumped on them. It can have as much of an effect on their emotions as the initial diagnosis of cancer. They have to revisit emotions they came to believe they moved beyond."

Vicki is emphatic when she says, "It's not unusual for someone to feel the incredible fear of what the lymphedema is and what it might mean. We need to help women 'normalize' the lymphedema, to make them realize it is not unique to them, bring it down to a common level."

Both Izetta and Vicki emphasize that recently there has been a huge change in the awareness of lymphedema. "In the last year," Vicki says, "there have been new approaches that put us leagues ahead of where we were."

"Yes," Izetta adds. "And I think if women learned after surgery that there was the possibility of lymphedema, they would take more care in trying to prevent it. It's sad that we had no resources until recently. When women came to us with lymphedema, we had nowhere to send them. Now we do. We still take the same care with them as we ever did. We try to draw them out, to help them get to a place where they can deal with the emotional issues—and believe me, there are some deep emotional issues with it."

Vicki and Izetta both agree that their task is to encourage women to talk about the feelings connected with the lymphedema, to explore not only the physical but the emotional effects of the swelling.

Izetta says, "We need to let women know they are not alone. Now there is help. We have to encourage them to demand help from their doctors. They must insist on seeing someone who is trained and experienced in the specific treatments for lymphedema—not just someone who does normal massage, but someone who knows how to do lymphatic massage."

Recent advances in the treatment and prevention of lymphedema indicate that education is extremely important.[2] Vicki agrees, saying that she thinks everyone who is being treated for breast cancer should be sent to a recognized lymphedema clinic. "As I've learned more about lymphedema, it occurs to me that women should be sent to physical therapy—or to some kind of class—to learn about lymphedema even *before* lymph node dissection."

Izetta concludes, "A women must not take 'No' for an answer. There is treatment available even if a woman's doctor doesn't know about it. She needs to insist that she get it. She is her own best advocate."

24

Ruth Bach: A Counselor Treats Herself and Others

RUTH BACH COUNSELS cancer patients. She also manages a cancer counseling center that treats dozens of cancer patients and their families each month. She is trim and fashionable, wearing a long, almost ankle-length skirt and black tunic.

She crosses her legs and settles in for our discussion. "I think," she says, "that depression is a response to the unendingness of things. In our society, we're geared for flight or fight. Depression can take the form of flight." Her observations come from her years of experience, almost three decades, spent counseling. "We depress ourselves so we don't feel the anxiety. Depression dulls the sharpness of our pain, gives us something to be part of. We are geared for resolution, and lymphedema is hard to resolve."

Ruth had been counseling women with breast cancer for seven years when her own breast cancer was diagnosed. "Knowing other women with breast cancer really helped me deal with my own cancer," she says. She had a lumpectomy, and lymph nodes were removed for staging. "I don't think I needed to have breast cancer to be a good counselor, but I feel it deepened my understanding—although I am also aware we are all individuals, that no two of us are alike. In each of us there are pockets, secret places, that no one will ever know or understand."

She speaks fast, without any preachiness or pomposity. "One of the greatest aids to survival," she says, "is having a sense of meaning and a sense that you belong to a community, a place where you have a connection. Health and recovery depend on it."

Her words come fast, as if she is eager to help every woman cope. "We have to speak up about our problems. We can't simply go on and"—she fingers quotes in the air—"'live with it' alone. It used to be the case with cancer. We were told we just had to live with it. It's now typical with lymphedema. Yes, you have to live with it, but that doesn't mean do nothing about it. Don't accept the 'There's nothing we can do' answer. If we are told there is nothing to be done, we need to ask, 'Then *who* can help me?' If you are not getting help or your questions aren't answered by your doctor, go to your cancer counselor, go to other cancer patients, call the advice nurses, talk to a physical therapist. There is help, but sometimes you need to search to find it."

She says that six years after her first bout with cancer, she had a recurrence. The second time she had a mastectomy and chemotherapy. "The second time there were no lymph nodes to remove. They had already been removed with the first operation."

After the second operation, Ruth developed lymphedema. She remembers precisely when it started. "It had been six years since the nodes were removed. For six years I had no problems at all. Then, not long after the second surgery, I was gardening, cutting up little limbs from a tree we had trimmed. Two days later," she holds out her right arm, which is slim and elegant, "my arm just ballooned. I think I was more upset with the swelling than I was at any time with the cancer. I was working in the medical community at that time, but no one knew about massage for swelling, or bandaging, or any of the techniques that are coming along now.

"On my own, I found a compression sleeve, and I wore that sleeve twenty-four hours a day for an entire year. It took a year, but the swelling did finally go away. Though," she massages a place on her arm just above the elbow, "there is still one little bump that hasn't gone away. I keep working at it. And I do this little mini-exercise." She shows how she pushes her fingers up her arm, moving toward her shoulder.

"It is normal," she says, "and healthy to be obsessive when something is wrong with you, particularly in the beginning. Sometimes obsession is our way of moving on. And it is healthy if, in the process, it helps you get through. Sometimes we *need* to focus, to obsess.

"I think often we push things away in our society. So pushing away, making the best of it, becomes our normal response. In order to take care of your body, you *have* to think about it. I think it's important to pay attention, in order to give yourself quality. Nothing matters without that. Self-esteem and ego are really important."

She holds out her arm again, tenderly strokes it. "For all practical purposes my lymphedema is gone. I use the tendons as my sign of whether it's swollen or not. I really watch to make sure I can still see them." She also adds that she works out with stationary weights and free weights. The free weights, she says, are not heavy, but she conscientiously does the repetitions. And she exercises every day. "If I don't do it every day I get little creaks and tingles. I don't know if they're in my imagination or not, but I don't like them. Sometimes I would love to take a vacation from the exercise drill." She laughs. "*Everybody* takes vacations. But I really can't. If I want to keep the swelling down, it's just something I am going to have to do forever."

She checks her watch, uncrosses her legs. She has an appointment soon. "One more thing," she says. "It occurs to me there are improvements in diagnosis coming along that are going to spare the lymph nodes in women in the future. And that is going to pose a dilemma for us who came before. I see that same dilemma in women who had the old-fashioned radical mastectomy." Her face grows stern. "Talk about deformity! Talk about immobility! I've had to counsel them and deal with their rage and their sorrow when they begin thinking they had cancer too early.

"We are going to experience that sorrow and regret ourselves one day. There *are* going to be improvements. Women in the future will not have to suffer as much as we do. And we must recognize and express our feelings about that. There has to be room for the protest. We have to let the two-year-old in us stamp her foot and scream. It doesn't make the pain go away, but it lets us honor ourselves and our experiences. We have to have room to say it."

25

The Powers of Mind and Spirit

FROM A HOLISTIC POINT OF VIEW, health and wellness include mental health and spiritual contentment as well as physical health and emotional well-being. In this chapter we look at the effects of stress on our lives and the potential benefits of relaxation, meditation, prayer, and visualization for people with lymphedema.

Dr. Chandler has seen the benefit to some of his patients who have reached out and begun incorporating nontraditional practices into their normal, recognized medical treatments. "In my practice, I'm encouraging people to strengthen their emotional, spiritual, and immune systems all together, to take everything into account: massage, walking, acupuncture, prayer. The benefits of all these things are becoming scientifically proven." Dr. Chandler laughs, then says, "Only in our country would we try to scientifically prove the effects of prayer. But some PET scans show improvement after prayer."

He also notes, "Our whole body does not respond well when we aren't taking care of ourselves, like the times when we don't eat right, or get enough rest or sleep."

As Dr. Chandler indicates, it is our "whole" self that gives us health, and finding that wholeness is the subject of this chapter. You may already be living some of what you'll find in this chapter. If so, good for you. If not, consider. The ideas are all geared toward healing, toward putting health first and making life fuller.

The Power of the Mind to Heal

Perhaps some of our most potent strengths lie in the power of our minds. Norman Cousins's story is well known and is told in his book, *Anatomy of an Illness as Perceived by the Patient.* Mr. Cousins wrote about his experience with a disease that was taking over his body, eating up the connective tissues in his spine and joints.[1] Sick in the hospital, with a life-threatening illness, Mr. Cousins began to think that sickness can come from thoughts, as much as from accident, trauma, disease, or hereditary disposition. He hypothesized that the reverse may also be true: if he could lighten his own mind, his body would follow.

He ordered film clips from *Candid Camera* to be sent to his room along with some old Marx brothers' films. And when he watched them, he started laughing.

The results were almost immediate. Ten minutes of belly laughs gave him two hours of pain-free sleep without any other painkillers. Even more important, the reductions were cumulative. After each session of laughter, his health continued to improve. He writes, "I have learned never to underestimate the capacity of the human mind and body to regenerate."[2]

If this technique of laughter and humor could prove so powerful in the case of Mr. Cousins' illness, what might it do to promote health in the case of lymphedema? Though there are no studies that prove the benefits of humor, how can it be anything but beneficial (and perhaps a little bit of fun as well)?

Relaxation and Stress

One way in which we can harness the power of our mind to heal is by becoming aware of how we handle stress. Our lives are filled with stress, and when we experience it, our body responds instantly: our muscles tense, we release adrenaline, our metabolism speeds up, we breathe faster, our blood sugar level rises, our heart speeds up, our blood pressure increases, and our blood supply is diverted from our stomach to our extremities. In other words, our body prepares us to fight or to flee.

In short spurts, stress serves an important purpose: it prepares us to respond to danger. But if stress becomes an ongoing part of our life, it can actually lower our body's immune response and can weaken, even damage, our systems. No one lives without stress, and knowing how to deal with stress can be an important ingredient in health. All of us have come down with a cold or the flu when we were under a great deal of stress. In fact, some of us who have had cancer felt it coming on during a particularly stressful time in our life. Some life events can especially ratchet up stress levels. Here is a short list of the most potent:[3]

- death of a spouse

- divorce

- marital separation

- serving a jail term

- death of a close family member

- personal injury or illness

- marriage

- being fired from a job

- marital reconciliation

- retirement

- change in the health of a family member

- pregnancy

- sexual difficulties

- gain of a new family member

- business readjustment

...and the list goes on.

Since you can't control everything outside you, your mission is to take charge of how you respond to it. Half the battle is realizing when stress has you in its grip. Be aware of times when your shoulders are pulling up toward your ears, your chest is tightening, you're clenching your teeth, or you're holding your breath or breathing faster.

Picture this: You are driving in heavy traffic. The traffic is making you late for a job interview for which you spent three days rewriting your resume. You are stopped dead at an intersection. Every time the light cycles from green to yellow to red your neck muscles cramp. Your fingers blanch, clutching the wheel. You are gritting your teeth, holding your breath. You are becoming a mess of tension, angry, scared that you'll miss out on a job that you imagine is the only job you'll ever have again in your life.

Will the tension you're storing up make the traffic move? Will you get to the interview any faster by holding your breath? What kind of interview will you have, anyway, if you get there feeling like you do?

Why not, right there in the midst of tailpipe exhaust, make a change? Why not unknot your stomach and give yourself a break?

Do this: Let your hands relax in your lap. Drop your shoulders and begin to breathe. Slowly inhale through your nose. Practice what you learned in the chapter on belly breathing. Allow your breath to go deep, to move only your stomach. Close your eyes. Whisper the breath out through your lips. Concentrate on letting go, on how you feel, on how much better the cramp in your neck is.

You have a choice. You can make yourself feel better. You will eventually get to the interview. How you feel when you get there is up to you.

Feeling better is the best part of relaxation, and feeling better is the product of a whole lot of physiological changes that relaxation brings about in our bodies. When we relax, our metabolism does an about-face from when it's stressed. Our blood pressure drops, our breathing slows, our muscles relax, and our metabolic rate decreases. It is a healthful state for us to be in. However, unlike the stress response, which can be triggered immediately, relaxation takes time and some focused effort to achieve.[4]

The list of tools that can help manage stress is long. Here, as with all of life, we need to experiment, to work until we learn what works for each of us. Some well-known options include:

- ◆ Engaging in regular exercise

- ◆ Practicing good nutrition

- ◆ Getting adequate sleep

- ◆ Minimizing emotional stressors (noisy environments, bright colors, extreme temperatures, strong smells, clutter, etc.)

- ◆ Surrounding yourself with people who support you (rather than drain you)

- ◆ Practicing belly breathing and pursuing progressive relaxation techniques

Relaxation and Prayer

Dr. Herbert Benson, head of the Mind/Body Medical Institute at Harvard Medical School and author of a book titled, *The Relaxation Response*, has studied the physiological effects of meditation, relaxation, and prayer for several years. In an article in the *New York Times* he is quoted as saying, "There are many activities you can use to evoke the relaxation response, yoga, meditation, running, music." But he goes on to add that about 80 percent of his patients choose prayer.[5] In other articles in *Prevention Magazine*, he says that to relax there are two basic steps to follow: the first is to break up thinking of everyday troubles. "One of the most effective ways to do this is through repetition: repeating a word, a sound, a thought, a breathing exercise or even a religious phrase."[4] He gives examples: "Christians might use 'Our Father who art in heaven,' Jews might choose, 'Shalom,' a Hindu might use 'Om.'" He says words like "peace," "calm," or "ocean" can work as well.[6]

The second step is to take time to relax *every day*—in fact, twice a day is best—and to do so for ten to twenty minutes. It can take a month to perfect the pattern, but soon your body will not respond to stress with as much ferocity as it once did.

Meditation and Visualization

We have known for a long time that there is a mind-body connection, but it is little understood and has been hard to document. Carl and Stephanie Simonton began to work with cancer patients in the early 1970s, using techniques of imagery and visualization in healing. Dr. Nicholas Hall of George Washington Medical Center in Washington, D.C., presented research in 1984 that demonstrated how a person's state of mind affects the immune system and how the immune system affects one's state of mind. Bernie Siegel, M.D., surgeon and author, expanded upon these ideas. In his book, *Love, Medicine, and Miracles,* he shares a great deal of information regarding the psychology of healing. In his work with exceptional cancer patients, healing has come about using techniques of relaxation, meditation, hypnosis, and visualization.[7]

Meditation is defined by Joan Borysenko, Ph.D., in her book *Minding the Body, Mending the Mind,* as "any activity that keeps the attention pleasantly anchored in the present moment."[8] Bernie Siegel feels it is a method by which one can "temporarily stop listening to the pressures and distractions of everyday life," and become more aware of "our deeper thoughts and feelings, the peace of pure consciousness, and spiritual awareness."[9]

Breathing is the initial focus in many forms of meditation— simply noticing the breath as it flows in and out. Some teachers recommend adding phrases and sounds that are meaningful to you: words and phrases such as "peace," "love," or "let go," sounds such as "mmmm" or "nnnn." Sometimes picturing a single, relaxing image works as well. Perhaps the image of a candle flame might work to calm you. It is important for you to pick your own word, sound, or image, choosing those that free your mind from its accustomed busy-ness and allow you to focus on *just being.*

As simple as this sounds, this settling in, this finding internal serenity, is difficult. It is contrary to our culture in which we are pressured to act, rewarded for keeping busy, so we find it hard to allow ourselves even short periods of inactivity and quiet.

Initially, people who consistently practice meditation find their concentration is improved. Continued practice gradually brings a sense of calmness, helping you to deal better with life's daily challenges. There is less of a stress response, and because of that, your emotional, mental, and physical well-being benefit. Bernie Siegel says, "I know of no other single activity that by itself can produce such great improvement in the quality of life."[10]

Visualization taps into a curious phenomenon: your body cannot distinguish between a vivid mental experience and an actual physical experience. There is now much documentation proving that you can cause a powerful physical response in your body through your mind's participation in visualization. Electromyographic studies of muscles have shown that simply imagining an activity will electrically activate the muscles that perform that activity.

Visualization is a technique that combines relaxation or meditation techniques with mental imagery. Guidelines for visualization include choosing your own image, and making it one that is realistic for you, one you can believe in and can see clearly in your mind's eye. Bernie Siegel notes that the Simontons made an initial misjudgment that all patients would respond to visualization involving fighting and warfare to kill their cancer cells. But many people were disturbed by mental imagery of warfare or killing and had difficulty relaxing with that image.

A more helpful visualization might be one in which the army of white blood cells is carrying the cancer cells away. Or, Dr. Siegel tells of a child who visualized his cancer as cat food and the immune cells as white cats.[11]

For someone with lymphedema, some suggestions for visualizations might include the following:

- See the existing healthy lymph vessels expanding, allowing lymph to flow out of the arm.

- Visualize little rivers of lymph flowing in new channels up and over the top of your shoulder, or across the midline of your body to a new quadrant.

- Visualize alternative pathways of flow that detour the impaired lymph system.

- Visualize the lymph nodes in other parts of your body pumping (the way we can imagine the heart pumping).

- Visualize each lymph angion, the single lymph vessel cell, pumping the next cell, and that one pumping the next, and the next, and so on.

- Focus on the one-way valves of the lymph vessels opening and then closing to prevent the backflow of lymph fluid.

- Focus on diaphragmatic breathing and visualizing the pressure changes in the thoracic cavity gently stimulating the central thoracic lymphatic duct in the area.

- See yourself with a smaller limb, and perhaps wearing clothes that demonstrate that.

- As you exercise against the bandage, visualize the lymph vessels being gently squeezed between the muscle and bandages, moving lymph fluid up your arm.

- Visualize your lymphatic massage assisting the flow of fluid.

Use your imagination to create any other visualizations that may have meaning for you. The choices are limitless.

When practicing visualization, your environment can become an aid as well. Surround yourself with whatever calms you and does not distract you: music, nature sounds, soft "white" noise. Some people find it helpful to make an audiotape to guide their visualizations, others prefer to do it themselves. To be most effective it is best to practice regularly over a period of several weeks. It is not realistic to practice once and expect significant results.

Practicing Visualization

To start, place yourself in a comfortable position, preferably sitting with your hands and feet uncrossed. Become aware of your breathing and the motion of your chest and abdomen. Slowly breathe in and out, noticing the gentle flow of air. Breathe in peacefulness and breathe out tension. Close your eyes if that is comfortable for you. Start at your forehead and gently work down through your body from head to your toes, one area at a time, focusing on each area, perhaps tightening and releasing. Notice the gradual release of tension as you move through your body. Your body may begin to feel heavy or warm.

Then picture a pleasant scene, one that is a safe place for you. Imagine the colors, aromas, and sounds. This is a place where wellness exists, your corner of the universe. Find a place to sit down in your scene. Take a few moments to just be there, taking time to allow the warmth of the sun and the energy of the earth to heal you. Here you are safe, and at peace.

Gradually notice the area of your body that is swollen with lymphedema. Visualize the lymph fluid leaving the area of your body where it has accumulated, and picture it flowing to new areas that can take care of it. Add whatever visualizations you think would be helpful now.

After spending several minutes with the visualizations you have chosen, let the awareness of your body begin to increase, perhaps noting the position you are in, the pressure of the chair against your back, the motion of your chest and abdomen as you breathe. Gradually notice yourself bringing your focus and attention back to the room.

To conclude the session, take several slow, deep, cleansing breaths, becoming more alert and awake with each breath. Allow yourself some quiet time to feel the benefits of this practice session before returning to your regular routine.

We can only scratch the surface of this topic here. There are many, many publications and tapes on it, both audio and video. Hundreds of practitioners are trained in visualization techniques, some leading classes. If you are interested, we encourage you to find a place where you can pursue this. Cancer counselors may be among your most valuable resources.

◆ ◆ ◆

Dr. Chandler says, "It is so important for all of us to discard that which clutters our lives. The media in this country seem obsessed by things that have little meaning. I feel that women must let go of some loads in their lives." He laughs. "Like letting go of emotional lymphedema." He continues, "Athletes aim to be in what they call The Zone, where outside and inside are absolutely one. The body is a healing machine, but you must let go sometimes as well. If everything is not perfect, if your edema continues, you are not a failure. You do the most you can, then you move on down the river."

Each of us is unique. Each of us finds peace and comfort in her own creative way. We must find what speaks to us in terms of health, peace, and power. Therein, for now, lies our journey. Feather's story exemplifies this journey. In the next chapter she relates how her discovery of physical as well as spiritual practice has helped her in the process of healing.

26

Feather: A Creative Approach to Healing

FEATHER HAS BEEN a psychiatric nurse for almost fifteen years. "I seem to have an affinity and appreciation for people with mental illness," she says. She finished her studies late in life, after her family was grown.

She is wearing a cotton tunic and loose, drapey slacks with an ornate Indian paisley design. Green earrings dangle from her ears. Her clothes are dramatic and say she is "with it"; she wears the sort of dress her grandchildren would appreciate. "I was diagnosed with cancer three years ago and I decided at the time I wasn't going to let it get the better of me. And I set to getting rid of it," she says. "The doctors wanted to dwell on statistics." She has blue eyes and a round face that even, in her early sixties, looks young. "But I am not a statistic. The mind is the most powerful organ in the body. The doctors couldn't know what I could do."

Feather had a mastectomy and reconstruction during the same operation. And she had to convince the surgeon to do it all at once. Her medical facility was not performing the procedures together at that time, so neither her surgeon nor her hospital had done them, though she knew other facilities were. She insisted that if her hospital did not do as she wanted she would find one that did. Her oncologist listened, and together they worked with the surgeon to do the operation as she wanted.

"I did so well and was feeling so good a couple of weeks after the surgery that I decided to redo the floor in my living room. I had no idea I needed to be careful about heavy, repetitive work, and after a couple of days my arm swelled way up. "I called my counselor in tears." She is animated as she says this. "I was just beginning to feel like I was living again and on the road to recovery. Then this swelling comes on. The counselor didn't have any idea what to suggest. I searched everywhere for help. My oncologist didn't know what to tell me. For two years I had lymphedema. I was crying out for help and no one knew how to help me."

She leans back, takes a breath. "Then I heard about people doing massage for lymphedema. My medical facility was not doing it, so my insurance didn't cover it. I was beginning to think I was going to have to fight again to make them give me a referral to an outside practitioner." She smiles. "As it turned out, because I was so insistent, my medical facility sent someone to training. I was my therapist's first patient. And the swelling started to subside."

She sits still a moment. The movement of her earrings goes quiet. "But it came back again. Last month I had surgery to loosen some of the scar tissue from my mastectomy. It became infected. My arm swelled again."

She holds out her arm. The lower part of it below her elbow is more swollen than her other arm.

"But I don't feel so panicked this time. I know what to do about it. I am sporadic about bandaging. I do it maybe once a week. But I do Qigong every morning," she says, "and am finding that it helps."

She says she learned Qigong from Master Chen Hui-Xien, who herself was diagnosed with a particularly virulent form of breast cancer fifteen years ago. The doctors told Chen Hui-Xien she had three, perhaps four, weeks to live. She refused to accept their prognosis and set out to search for a cure and rehabilitation for herself. She discovered a form of Qigong she called Soaring Crane.

"Qigong means life-breath, life-work, energy," Feather says.

"Breathing oxygenates your body. Qigong is as ancient as Tai Chi. But it is not like Tai Chi, which is a martial art. Qigong is strictly for healing and health. It teaches breathing and visualizing to bring in the universal energy. You learn to exhale in ways that rid your body of the disease." She waves her arms gently over her head. Her movements are quiet, dance-like, stylized. "Like a soaring crane," she says.

"I was real sick when I was in chemotherapy. But every morning, or almost every morning, I went to a special garden near a mansion in town. The garden was hidden behind a forest of trees. There, before anyone was up, I breathed and did Qigong. I always came home feeling better. I think Qigong is why my lymphedema is not too bad anymore, even after the infection.

"These last three years have been a gift for me, really." She strokes one of the earrings, seems to gain peace from it. "I feel an opportunity for aliveness. My connections with people are so much deeper. Everything has deepened; the spiritual, the reason to be alive."

She sets her hands together in her lap. "I have learned to be very, very kind—kind with my surgeons, kind with my therapist, with all the people working with me. I have compassion for them. I wanted them involved in my healing, and I feel these kinds of thoughts have helped everyone work better on me." She tips her head back, laughs. "Though I'll tell you, I wasn't going to let anybody cut on me who I didn't know."

She is quiet again, the earrings still. "I feel so blessed, so unafraid now. I have an opportunity to be on the path of gratitude. Once I decided I really wanted to live, it was like infinite connections came: new friends, fascinating learning, energy."

27

Nutritional Supplements

As we've seen in previous sections of the book and in several of the stories, sometimes resources beyond the traditional treatments can help tremendously. This includes diet as well as some emerging nutritional resources that are showing promise in benefiting lymphedema. Here is a summary of some of them.

Flavonoids

Flavonoids are also known as Vitamin P, and occur naturally in many foods. Blueberries are rich in flavonoids, as are onions, apples, green tea, and the pith of citrus fruits. You can also buy flavonoids in health food stores throughout the country, but usually they are mixed with other nutrients and sold as *bioflavonoids*.

Dr. Judith Casley-Smith, who works with the Lymphoedema Association of Australia, says flavonoids work slowly—it may take months to be able to measure a reduction in swelling—but can be effective. Flavonoids are made up of large molecules and thus are quite bulky for the body to absorb. Because only a small part of the molecule is effective for lymphedema, dosages must be high (3,000 to 6,000 mg/day).[1] Complicating the dose requirement is the fact that the flavonoids normally found in the stores are mixed with other nutrients. Most bioflavonoid complexes yield only 50 percent flavonoids.

Flavonoids can upset your stomach, so if you decide to try them start with smaller dosages and let your body adjust before you work up to a level that will reduce the swelling.

Pycnogenols

Pycnogenols are also bioflavonoids. European physicians have known since 1950 that Pycnogenols strengthen capillaries and reduce swelling in legs and ankles.[2] Pycnogenol is a trade name, and the company that manufactures Pycnogenols insists the only real source is the bark of the French maritime pine.[3] In truth, the same chemical composition is also found (somewhat cheaper) in grape seeds. You can find them both in health food stores.

Pycnogenols have no known toxic side effects. They work synergistically with Vitamin C to reinforce Vitamin C's function in capillary membranes and in strengthening collagen in the capillaries.[3] Recommended dosages differ, depending on body weight and on how long you have been taking them.[4]

Selenium

Though, in the past, Selenium was thought to improve the efficacy of decongestive lymphatic therapy by as much as 10 percent,[5] no research supports this. However, some people still believe it may have benefits in blocking oxidation radicals and affecting an anti-inflammatory reaction. Good sources for selenium are Brazil nuts, eggs, lean meats, seafood, legumes, and whole grains.[6] Selenium can, however, be toxic, and it is recommended that you discuss its use with your physician before taking it.[7]

The Benzo-pyrones

The most common compounds used to treat lymphedema belong to the chemical family called the benzo-pyrones. The smallest of these and the base molecule is called Coumarin. Benzo-pyrones have been used with success in treating lymphedema in Australia, India, England, and elsewhere,[7] but the jury may still be out on their effectiveness. A recent study in the *New England Journal of Medicine* found that Coumarin had no effect in a group of 140 women with chronic lymphedema.[8] Dr. Casley-Smith reports that her research shows that Coumarin is slow-acting, taking weeks or months to work. It may be taken in three ways: orally, or applied in powders, or in creams. Though benzo-pyrones are undergoing trials in the United States, the FDA has not yet approved them. And, as a word of caution, the oral application has been deregistered in Australia because a small percentage of patients experienced a type of hepatitis. This liver problem seems to resolve when the benzo-pyrones are discontinued.[7]

Coumarin works by building the body's supply of macrophages. Macrophages break down and consume waste cells and high-protein edemas.[7] As they work, protein molecules, waste cells, viruses, and bacteria in the areas of swelling are reduced and the possibility increases for the body to develop alternative pathways to remove the buildup of protein.

No side effects have been reported from the topical uses of Coumarin, except an occasional mild skin allergy, which goes away if applications are discontinued.[7]

It has recently become possible to purchase benzo-pyrones in the United States, but doing so requires a prescription from your doctor. Here are some suggestions as to where you can get them:

J. R. Hadfield, R.Ph.
Hadfield's Pharmacy
21701 76th Avenue W., Suite 104
Edmonds, WA 98026
Tel.: (206) 744-1799; Fax: (206) 744-1797

B. Bradshaw, R.Ph.
Custom Care Pharmacy
6103 Johns Road, Suite #1
Tampa, FL 33634
Tel.: (800) 995-4363; (813) 822-4500; (813) 882-0201

Mr. S. Nagy, C.P.T., M.P.
Total Care Pharmacy
5905 Hampton Oaks Parkway, Suite C
Tampa, FL 33610

Tel.: (800) 424-0920; (813) 621-4800
Fax: (800) 835-9935; (813) 622-7939

Barry Smith
Medical Dental Pharmacy
6327 N. Fresno
Fresno, CA 93710
Tel.: (800) 794-2832; (559) 439-1190
Fax: (559) 439-1655

Miscellaneous Nutritional Compounds

An article in the July 1996 newsletter of the National Lymphedema Network[9] mentions several holistic nutritional supplements that may help in patients' self-care. While the National Lymphedema Network says it does not endorse these supplements, they still present the alternatives as something for us to consider.

Inflamzyme Forte. This is a combination of digestive enzymes designed to reduce the accumulation of fats and proteins in the lymphatic system. Inflamzyme Forte has similar effects to benzo-pyrones, but no side effects.

Lymphotend. Lymphotend works in combination with Inflamzyme Forte. It is a homeopathic remedy that the Bradford Institute in Chula Vista, California, is researching.

Horsechestnut Herb. Horsechestnut herb has been found to be as effective as compression garments for treating chronic diseases of the veins.

Vitamins, minerals, antioxidants. The National Lymphedema Network (NLN) encourages the use of good multiple vitamins along with potent antioxidants (like the Pycnogenols). The NLN recommends specific manufacturers—for example, Phyto Pharmica, Enzymatic Therapies, AMNI, Solgar, and Twin Labs.

Part Four

Finding Resources

28

Where to Get Help

SLOWLY, GROUPS ARE EMERGING that specialize in the problems associated with lymphedema. Here is a listing of some of them to consider in your search for information, therapists, services, or networks of people with lymphedema.

The National Lymphedema Network
2211 Post Street, Suite 404
San Francisco, CA 94115-3427
Info line: (800) 541-3259; Direct line: (415) 921-1306
Web site: www.lymphnet.org
Email: NLN@Lymphnet.org

The National Lymphedema Network is a nonprofit organization founded in 1988 by Saskia R. J. Thiadens, R.N. The organization provides education and guidance to lymphedema patients, health care professionals, and the general public. The NLN is supported by tax-deductible donations. Here are some of the services it provides:

◆ Referral to lymphedema treatment centers and health care professionals. The Network lists therapists certified to perform treatment for lymphedema. Not all therapists register with the NLN, and there may be additional qualified therapists in your area.

◆ Quarterly newsletters with information about medical and scientific developments, support groups, pen pals, updated resource guides, and more.

◆ Educational courses for health care professionals and patients.

◆ An extensive computer database.

◆ Biennial international conferences.

Lerner Lymphedema Services
Main office: Lymphedema Services, P.C.
245 E. 63rd Street, #106
New York, NY 10032
Tel.: (800) 848-1015; (212) 688-6107
Lerner Lymphedema Services also have offices in:
Boston, MA   Tel.: (617) 367-6162
New Brunswick, NJ   Tel.: (800) 882-9498
Sunrise, FL   Tel.: (800) 232-5542; (954) 846-7855
Web site is www.lymphedemaservices.com.

Lerner Lymphedema Services has a team of board-certified physicians and specially trained therapists who treat lymphedema and its complications. Robert Lerner, MD, F.A.C.S., is the medical director. Lerner Lymphedema Services makes available two clear, concise videos on remedial exercises to treat lymphedema. Order the videos through the New York office listed above. To schedule a consultation or to receive additional information, you can contact any of the four offices mentioned above.

Academy of Lymphatic Studies
12651 W. Sunrise Blvd
Sunrise, FL 33323
Tel.: (800) 232-5542
Web site: www.lymphedemaservices.com
Email: lymphdoc@bridge.net

The Academy of Lymphatic Studies offers an extensive training program for lymphedema, including training of medical doctors, physical therapists, nurses, occupational therapists, and massage therapists (if the massage therapists have fulfilled certain criteria for entry). The Academy of Lymphatic Studies also maintains a listing and reference service of therapists in their program.

Lymphedema Therapy Center Casley-Smith Method
770 Old Roswell Place, Suite I-400
Roswell, GA 30076
Tel.: 770-518-4700
Director: DeCourcy Squire, PT, CLT

The Lymphedema Therapy Center treats patients who have lymphedema or other disorders of the lymphatic system.

The Lymphoedema Association of Australia
94 Cambridge Terrace
Malvern, SA 5061
Australia
Tel.: +61(8) 8271-2198; Fax: +61(8) 8271-8776
Web site: http://www.lymphoedema.org.au
Email: Casley@enternet.com.au

This group is a leader in worldwide research and treatment of lymphedema. The Lymphoedema Association of Australia was formed by doctors John R. and Judith R. Casley-Smith in 1982. Its mission is to perform research, to aid patients, and to educate patients, therapists, and doctors. The LAA has also been a leader in research and education on the use and benefits of decongestive lymphatic therapy, and the effect of benzo-pyrones on lymphedema. The LAA can make available a library of pamphlets, videos, and newsletters. Their most recent publications include *Modern Treatment for Lymphoedema*, and *High-Protein Oedemas and the Benzo-Pyrones* (for doctors and therapists), *Information About Lymphoedema for Patients*, and *Exercises for Patients with Lymphoedema of the Arm and a Guide to Self-Massage and Hydrotherapy*. They also have music tapes to accompany the exercise routines, as well as videos on exercises, causes of edema, benzo-pyrones, and microcirculation. Write or email for prices.

Dr. Vodder Schule-Walchsee
Alleestrasse 30, A-6344 Walchsee
Tyrol, Austria
Tel.: +43-5374-5245-0; Fax: +43-5374-5245-4
Web site: www.vodderschule.com
Email: vodder@fx.tirol.netwing.at

The Vodders pioneered the manual lymph drainage system. In 1967 the Society for Dr. Vodders' Manual Lymph Drainage (MLD®) was founded. The society's aim was to scientifically substantiate the effect of MLD® and to create courses of study for various professional groups. The Vodder School maintains lists of Vodder-certified therapists throughout the world.

Dr. Vodder School of North America
P.O. Box 5701
Victoria, B.C., V8R 6S8
Canada
Tel. (250) 598-9862; Fax: (250) 598-9841
Web site: www.vodderschool.com
Email: drvodderna@vodderschool.com

This is the North American branch of the Dr. Vodder School. Robert Harris directs the school, which offers training programs for therapists throughout Canada and the United States and can provide information about MLD®-certified therapists in your area.

The North American Vodder Association of Lymphatic Therapy (NAVALT)
Tel.: (888) 4NAVALT ([888] 462-8258)
Fax: 972-243-3227

The North American Vodder Association of Lymphatic Therapy can provide lists of therapists certified in North America by the Dr. Vodder School.

The Foeldi Clinic
   Clinic of Lymphology
   Rosslehofweg 2-6
   79856 Hinterzarten
   Germany
   Tel.: +49-7652-1240; Fax: +49-7652-124315

The Foeldi Clinic was started in the early 1980s. It trains occupational and physical therapists, massage therapists, physicians, and nurses. Recently it has added classes geared to English-speaking therapists and to physicians.

The Foeldi Clinic also offers intensive residential treatment programs for people with lymphedema.

Lymphatic Therapy Associates
   1800 N.W. Market Street, Suite 201
   Seattle, WA 98107-3908
   Tel.: (206) 784-6988

Lymphatic Therapy Associates makes available two videotapes. One of these, *Self-Care for Post Mastectomy Lymphedema*, offers a step-by-step maintenance and prevention program for patients who have had mastectomies, lumpectomies, and/or axillary lymph dissections, and others at risk for developing lymphedema. The other video is *Lower Extremity Lymphedema*. Ms. Rovig is an experienced lymphedema practitioner who has developed these tapes to provide an overview of what lymphedema is, and instruction for self-massage and bandaging. They are not meant to be a substitute for lymphedema care but an adjunct to a comprehensive care program provided by a trained therapist.

Lyphedema Therapy
    7 Froehlich Farm Blvd.
    Woodbury, Long Island, NY 11797
    Tel.: (516) 364-2200
    Fax: (516) 364-1844
    Marvin Boris, M.D.
    Bonnie B. Lasinski, P.T.

Physicians and physical therapists at Lymphedema Therapy have been trained in Complex Lymphedema Therapy (CLT) by Dr. John Casley-Smith and Dr. Judith Casley-Smith of Australia. The practice is dedicated to the diagnosis, treatment, and management of individuals with both primary and secondary lymphedema, including lymphedema complicated by open wounds. Patient education and self care are emphasized.

Other Internet Addresses
    For support groups: www.wenet/lymphnet
    Lymphedema International network: www.lymphedema.com
    Search "lymphedema" on the Web at: oncolink.upenn.edu

29

When You Are Seeking Treatment

WHEN YOU OR YOUR DOCTOR decide it is time to treat your lymphedema, you'll face many issues not only in the search for treatment but in getting it paid for. In this chapter we will make some suggestions on getting treatment for lymphedema as well as discuss insurance coverage.

Questions to Ask When Considering Treatment[1]

Here is a list of questions you can use as a guideline for what you might want to ask when you are seeking answers and deciding on treatment. They are based on those suggested by the National Lymphedema Network, but be sure to get all your own questions answered as well.

The Program

What kind of programs do you offer? Do they include manual lymphatic drainage or something comparable?

Would you use continuous compression during or after my therapy? If so, what kind (bandages, garments, etc.)?

How long is your program? If I need longer treatment, would you provide it?

Do I need authorization from my doctor to begin treatment?

How much training do your therapists have? (Note: The United States has not set standards. In Europe, the minimum training to be certified is 135 to 150 hours.)

What results can I expect?

Can I contact and get a recommendation from someone who has been through your program?

Products

Do you sell bandages and compression garments, or do you have recommendations for where I can buy them?

Are you qualified to measure me for garments, or is the place you recommend qualified to do the measurements?

Care After Treatment

Will you train me to manage my lymphedema after treatment? Will you educate me in areas such as self-massage, skin care, exercise regimens, diet, and complementary holistic therapies?

Do you have a lymphedema support group, or do you know of one in the area?

Do you provide emergency assistance, or help on holidays, weekends, and evenings?

Costs

How much does the program cost?

When will I pay for treatment?

Can you bill my insurance company? If so, do I need a preauthorization before I begin treatment?

Is there a cost for follow-up treatment?

Insurance

Resistance on the part of insurance companies to cover lymphedema continues to be a real problem. Only in the last year has the armor begun to crack. Since insurance normally covers only conditions and diseases that have been studied scientifically and have undergone clinical trials, and since the treatment of lymphedema has not been the subject of such trials, the insurance companies have refused to pay for treatment, maintaining there is no proof that it works.[2] In fact, nothing but pumps and sometimes garments have been covered by insurance, and use of them is no longer considered standard protocol. So where does that leave us?

Until recently, to be treated, we had to pay out of our own pockets. In much of the country that is still the case. However, as we have mentioned, there is mounting pressure for change. In the last ten years, some insurance companies have begun to realize that lymphedema, when left untreated, can lead to serious and expensive complications. This has provided some of the impetus for change.

The government includes lymphedema in its ICD-9 (International Classification of Diagnosis) codes. This is the diagnostic coding system insurance companies and the medical community use to describe conditions, surgeries, and diseases. The 1999 edition of the CPT (Current Procedural Terminology) manual establishes a new code, #97140, which reads, "Manual therapy techniques (e.g., mobilization/manipulation, manual lymph drainage (lymphatic massage), manual traction), one or more regions, each 15 minutes."

The CPT manual is published by the American Medical Association and the codes are used to describe treatment procedures when billing to insurance companies.[3] This may open the door for the medical community to be reimbursed by insurance companies for treatment of lymphedema.

Change may be coming from other fronts as well. In October 1997, Medicare in Florida began covering costs for lymphedema treatment as long as the treatment is prescribed by a doctor as a medical necessity.[2]

In April 1997, Senator Edward Kennedy introduced bill S-609, which passed the Senate and in May was referred to the House of Representatives. The bill would approve the costs of complications from mastectomy, including lymphedema.[4] During the last part of 1998, President Clinton signed Public Law 105-227, the Women's Health and Cancer Rights Act of 1998. The law expands coverage for mastectomies and related services to include all stages of reconstructive surgery; surgery and reconstruction to produce a symmetrical appearance; prostheses; and treatment of physical complications, *including lymphedema.*

In the meantime, what can you do?

First, call your insurance company and ask about treatment. As we said, a few companies do cover lymphedema. If it is covered, be sure you find out which therapists or practitioners the policy covers. Find out, as well, if there is a deductible or co-payment. Ask if they cover in-patient or out-patient care, and if they pay for future, ongoing treatment.

Be prepared to provide your insurance company with documentation about the effectiveness of treatment and the consequences of leaving your lymphedema untreated. Copy articles from the National Lymphedema Network's newsletter. Go to your library and find journals that support your stance. Show them this book.

Ask questions of providers. Don't be embarrassed to question potential therapists about their background and training.[1] Some insurance carriers or HMOs will only pay for care from someone who is listed in their plans as a preferred provider (or someone employed directly by them). If your insurance carrier does not have anyone trained or certified in decongestive lymphatic therapy, request a referral to someone outside the system. All insurance carriers have some kind of mechanism for covering outside service if it is not provided in-house.

Involve your doctor. She or he may have suggestions and strategies that can help get your insurance company to cover treatment. Phrases such as "manual lymph drainage," "lymphatic mobilization," "bandaging," and "exercise," are usually more acceptable to insurance companies than "massage," which is not as likely to be covered.

Involve your therapist. Sometimes the lines between lymphedema and other conditions are blurred. If lymphedema is not the only condition for which you need treatment, perhaps your therapist can treat your lymphedema along with your other condition, which might be covered under your policy.

Point out the high costs that may be incurred by the insurance company from possible complications if your lymphedema is left untreated. Mention the potential for infections, skin disorders, and even hospitalization. Treatment for a single infection could equal the cost of lymphedema treatment.

Document your contacts with your insurance carrier. Each time you speak with them, be sure to note the name of the person you speak with and the date and time you talk. Keep copies of letters you send them along with copies of any information you've included.

Until the seriousness of lymphedema is recognized and the need for up-to-date treatment is accepted, you will need to act as your own advocate. You may want to consider writing Senator Kennedy in support of Senate bill S-609. Though it was introduced in 1997, the bill was still languishing in committee at the time this book went to print. Educate your doctor. Form or join a support group with others who are grappling with the problem of lymphedema. Who knows—maybe your efforts will be just the thing to push the system into action and get us the help we all know we need.

30

Conclusion

WE HOPE THE INFORMATION in this book helps answer the dozens of questions you might have about lymphedema. We hope it helps give you a sense of control over your future, and a sense that there is a community of us—millions, in fact—who know intimately what you are going through. We hope it helps you deal with your doctors and with your therapists. Writing it has been truly illuminating for both of us.

Note from Gwen

Writing this book has been a tremendous experience for me— helping me to grow as a therapist, making me learn everything I could about lymphedema, and challenging me as I wrote and worked with patients. I have decided one of the best ways to learn something is to do as much research as you can, then try to understand it and simplify it in order to present and teach it to someone else.

In the past year, I have seen many advances taking place in the study and treatment of lymphedema. There have been many more professional journal publications and books. More research on lymphedema is being carried out all over the world every week. There are many more therapists trained to work with it, and there is an increase in lymphedema treatment programs as well as a slowly increasing awareness and openness of doctors to refer their patients with lymphedema to those treatment programs. Legislation is being passed, paving the way for insurance coverage of lymphedema treatment as a complication of breast cancer. We are moving in the right direction.

I still feel blessed every day to be able to work with people who have lymphedema. It is an enriching experience for me and one that I am grateful to have. While I do not personally have lymphedema, or know its challenges firsthand, I am very empathetic with those who do. I have a strong desire to help, to teach, and to empower people to take care of themselves. It is my hope that this book will provide you with some tools you can put to use immediately, and that it can start you on the path of healing.

Note from Jeannie

This is my last chance for a personal update before the book goes to print. After nearly a year of being good about my daily home treatments and maintenance, I lapsed. I rebelled. For several months, I did nothing about my arm, and it swelled, gaining over an inch in some places.

Well, once that experiment (tantrum, really) was finished, I went back to dealing with it. I lost seven or eight pounds. I started wearing a garment most of the time (even at night) and bandaging whenever I do extra-hard work. I doubled my walking each week from ten to twelve miles to twenty to twenty-five. I do a short massage and breathing routine every day, and I started teaching an exercise/dance class that emphasizes arm movements and breathing. And, I began taking Coumarin. Three months later, my arm is about where it was when I was so good. So much for tantrums, at least for now. I've learned so much, not only about lymphedema but also about my own ability to slog through adversity to regain enjoyment in life.

All of us who have lymphedema will need to deal with it for the rest of our lives. What each of us decides to do about it is up to us. We don't choose to have lymphedema, but we don't choose to have cavities in our teeth either; so we floss, and we eat our spinach and our servings of fruit, and we make other efforts to maintain ourselves and do the best we can with our lives. And so it is with lymphedema. Lymphedema is simply something that requires our care. The better we attend to it as part of our overall health, the more we can resume and enjoy the things we love. Isn't that the way with everything in life?

Again we must thank a handful of people for the knowledge we now have about lymphedema: the Vodders, who developed the first treatments; the Foeldis, who brought the techniques further into the world's view; Drs. John R. and Judith Casley-Smith, whose Lymphoedema Association of Australia conducts worldwide research and education; Saskia Thiadens, who has dedicated years to championing lymphedema education and has provided a system for us to communicate by founding the National Lymphedema Network in the United States; and Dr. Robert Lerner, whose system of clinics trains practitioners and treats patients. Help is at our fingertips. We need only reach out for it to make life productive and worth living again.

Glossary

Abdomen The section of the body between the chest and the pelvis.

Acupuncture Traditional Chinese medicine involving insertion of thin needles into the body at specific locations.

Adjuvant Term used to describe an auxiliary treatment. In cancer, this is chemotherapy, radiation, or hormone therapy that is used to control, destroy, or reduce cancer cells that may have migrated to other areas of the body.

Aerobic Living in the presence of oxygen, as with aerobic exercise, which makes the heart and lungs work harder to meet the muscles' need for oxygen.

Angion A single vessel (such as a lymph vessel) that lies between two adjacent valves.

Antibiotics Drugs or other substances that destroy or inhibit the growth of microorganisms.

Antibodies Protein molecules made by the lymph system that fight bacteria, viruses, or other foreign bodies.

Antioxidants Substances that inhibit reactions promoted by oxygen. It is believed that antioxidants play a role in preventing or slowing the growth of some types of cancer.

Arterial Pertaining to the arteries.

Arterial capillaries The smallest blood vessels carrying blood from the heart.

Artery A large blood vessel that carries blood with oxygen from the heart to the rest of the body.

Atrophy Reduction in size of a cell, tissue, organ, or part of the body due to a failure of nutrition to that part.

Axilla The space under the shoulder between the upper part of the arm and the side of the chest (also called the armpit).

Axillae Plural of Axilla.

Axillary node dissection Surgical procedure involving the removal of lymph nodes in the armpit.

B-Cell A type of white blood cell, also called a lymphocyte, that plays a role in the body's immune response.

B-Lymphocytes See B-Cell.

Bandaging In treatment of lymphedema, the application of a series of wraps that have a special low-stretch property (as opposed to Ace bandages, which are high-stretch).

Belly See Abdomen.

Benzo-pyrones Compounds that stimulate the body's immune system to help remove stagnant protein in the body's tissue, helping to reduce lymphedema. Also called Coumarin or Lodema. Not currently approved by the FDA.

Bilateral mastectomy Removal of both breasts.

Bioflavonoids Also called Vitamin P. Bioflavonoids are necessary in the absorption of Vitamin C.

Biologic Relating to life and living things. In medicine, a product used in the prevention or treatment of disease

Breast conservation surgery Surgical treatment for breast cancer that removes only the tumor, tissue around the tumor, and axillary lymph nodes. Also called lumpectomy, segmental mastectomy.

Capillaries The smallest blood vessels which link the arteries and the veins.

Cardiovascular Having to do with the heart and the blood vessels.

CAT scan See CT scan.

Cellulitis Infection of the skin or subcutaneous tissue. Symptoms are heat, redness, pain, and swelling.

Chemotherapy The treatment of disease using highly toxic drugs given intravenously or orally.

Chest cavity The space inside the chest.

Chest wall The area on the trunk above the abdomen and below the collarbone consisting of the sternum and ribs.

Circulatory system The system of blood, blood vessels, lymphatics, and heart related to the circulation of blood and lymph.

Collateral Accessory or secondary, not direct, such as small access vessels.

Collateral lymph vessels Secondary or small branches of the lymph vessels that connect lymph quadrants.

Collecting Vessels Vessels in the lymphatic system that the lymph capillaries drain into.

Complication A secondary disease or condition that develops in the course of a primary disease or condition.

Complete physical therapy (CPT) Also called complex decongestive physiotherapy (CDP), or combined physiotherapy; now usually called decongestive lymphatic therapy. Therapy used to treat lymphedema. It includes meticulous skin care, lymphatic massage known as manual lymph drainage (MLD®), compression using special bandages, and garments, and exercise.

Compression garment A tightly knit elastic stocking or sleeve that, when worn, applies pressure to an area of the body to prevent fluid from flowing back and accumulating in the limb.

Compression pump See Vasopneumatic pump.

Compression therapy See Bandaging.

Compromised When used with reference to physical systems, those that are endangered or not working at optimal capacity.

Congenital Present from birth.

Congestive heart failure A condition in which there is an abnormal accumulation of fluid around the heart.

Constriction A tightening, as in to make narrower.

Contraction A shortening or development of tension, as in muscular contraction.

Contraindication Any condition that renders a treatment improper or undesirable.

Contralateral Pertaining to the opposite side.

Cosmetic Beautifying, to preserve beauty; made for the sake of appearance.

Coumarin See Benzo-pyrones.

CT scan Computerized axial tomography. A computerized X-ray that produces a highly detailed cross-sectional picture of the body.

Decongestive therapy Therapy that reduces the accumulation of fluid in the tissues.

Diaphragm A muscular partition or membrane separating the chest and the abdominal cavities.

Diaphragmatic breathing Breathing in which the diaphragm contracts, and moves up and down. Sometimes referred to as belly breathing or abdominal breathing. It is believed this type of breathing aids in the movement of lymph.

Dicloxacillan An antibiotic especially effective in treating skin infections.

Distal Farthest from the point of attachment or origin; for example, the elbow is distal to the shoulder.

Diuretics Drugs or other substances that promote the formation and release of urine.

Edema   The presence of abnormally large amounts of fluid in the tissue spaces of the body.

Edematous   Having edema.

Electromyographic   A method that tests electrical potential of muscle and records nerve and muscle function.

Enzymes   Complex proteins that are capable of accelerating or producing specific biochemical reactions at body temperature.

Ethyfoam roller   A Styrofoam-like roll two to four feet long and four to six inches in diameter, used in exercise.

Familial   Occurring in or affecting different members of the same family.

Fibrosclerotic   Fibers becoming hardened in tissues.

Fibrosis   The spreading of fiberlike connective tissue over normal, smooth muscle or other tissue.

Fibrotic   Having to do with fibrosis; harder than normal tissue, often referred to as scar tissue.

Filariasis   Infestation of the lymphatics by a mature larvae of a parasite, *Wuchereria bancrofti*.

Filter   Strain water or other fluid to separate out particulate matter.

Filtration   Outflowing of fluids in the body, as when blood and its components filter into interstitial tissues through arterial capillaries.

Flavonoids   Having to do with flavones, crystalline compounds found in many plants. Flavonoids are believed to aid in the processing of proteins, bacteria, and other foreign matter in the body.

Genetic   Pertaining to birth or origin, inherited.

Gymnastic ball   A large ball used in performing exercises particularly to gain and maintain strength and flexibility.

Hypoallergenic Not likely to cause an allergic response.

Immune system The body's ability to protect itself from disease, organisms, other foreign bodies, and cancers. The lymphatic system is a part of the immune system.

Immunity The capacity to resist a disease, organism, other foreign body, or cancer.

Indication That which indicates the proper treatment. A circumstance that shows the cause, pathology, or treatment of a disease.

Inflammation A response by the body to cells damaged by injury or irritation. The signs of inflammation are usually redness, pain, heat, and swelling.

Initial lymph vessels The fingerlike projections into the interstitial tissue where the lymph enters the lymphatic system; the beginning of the lymph system.

In situ Confined to the site of origin without invading neighboring tissues.

Interstitial The space between the body's tissues.

Interventions Actions intended to prevent an occurrence or maintain or alter a condition.

Invasive breast cancer Breast cancer that has spread into the breast tissue.

Involved limb The arm or leg that has lymphedema.

Involved quadrant The lymphatic drainage quarter of the body that has lymphedema.

Keflex The trademark name for an antibiotic that is particularly effective in treating infections of the skin.

Kyphotic thoracic spine Curvature of the thoracic spine from the lower cervical area to the upper lumbar. Characterized by vertebra with ribs attached.

Lumpectomy Surgical removal of a breast tumor, a small area of surrounding tissue, and some axillary lymph nodes. Also called breast conservation surgery.

Lymph A thin, pale, clear, yellowish fluid that bathes the body's tissues, passes into lymphatic channels and ducts, and is filtered by the lymph nodes before it is discharged into the blood by way of the thoracic duct.

Lymphangiography X-ray examination of the lymph glands and vessels after injection of a dye.

Lymphangiosarcoma A rare cancer of the lymphatic system.

Lymphangitis A bacterial infection of the lymphatic system.

Lymphatic capillary Small vessel carrying lymph.

Lymphatic massage Special very gentle massage that stimulates the lymphatic system and moves fluid from an area of the body that is unable to process it to an area that can. Also called manual lymph drainage.

Lymphatics Having to do with lymph, tissue relating to the lymph glands, lymph vessels, or lymphocytes.

Lymphatic system A vast and complex network of capillaries, thin vessels, valves, ducts, and nodes that is responsible for returning excess fluid from the tissues to the heart, which returns it to the blood. Also plays a role in protecting the body against illness.

Lymphatic vessels Vessels that convey lymph.

Lymphedema Swelling caused by an accumulation of lymphatic fluid in the tissues.

Lymphedema, congenital Lymphedema that is present from birth.

Lymphedema, praecox Primary lymphedema that develops during adolescence.

Lymphedema, primary Lymphedema that has no known cause.

Lymphedema, secondary Lymphedema that occurs after compromise to the lymphatic system by surgery, trauma, radiation, or infection.

Lymphedema, tarda Primary lymphedema that develops in adulthood, usually after the age of thirty-five.

Lymph nodes Small oval structures that remove waste from the body's tissues, filter lymph, fight infection, and produce white blood cells. There are five hundred to fifteen hundred lymph nodes, usually clumped in groups in the neck, axilla, groin, abdomen, and trunk.

Lymphocytes Special small white blood cells that increase in number and customize themselves to destroy foreign protein and to fight infections.

Lymphology The study of lymphatics.

Lymphoscintigraphy A diagnostic technique that creates a two-dimensional picture of lymph vessels by using radioisotopes.

Macrophages Large wandering cells that ingest microorganisms or other cells and foreign particles.

Malfunction Dysfunction.

Malignancy Cancerous growth.

Mammary glands Glands pertaining to the breast.

Manual lymph drainage (MLD®) A special massage technique that transports lymphatic fluid from an area of congestion or edema to an area of the body with functioning lymphatics. Used to treat lymphedema.

Mastectomy Surgical removal of one breast, tissue, and lymph nodes in the axilla on the same side. Also known as modified radical mastectomy.

Metabolism The chemical change in living cells by which energy is provided for vital processes.

Metastasis The spread of cancer cells to distant parts of the body, usually through the lymph system or blood vessels.

Microbes A minute organism or bacteria. A germ.

Milroy's disease Form of hereditary lymphedema, present at birth, in which there is an absence of initial lymph vessels.

MLD® See **Manual lymph drainage.**

MRI Magnetic resonance imaging. Test using electromagnets, frequency waves, and computer to provide an image.

Muscle hyperactivity Excessive activation of muscles.

National Lymphedema Network (NLN) The main clearinghouse of information on lymphedema in the United States.

Nodes See Lymph nodes.

Oncologist A doctor specializing in the study and treatment of cancer.

Oncology The study of cancer and its treatment.

Oxygenate To saturate with oxygen.

Pain threshold The point at which pain receptors are stimulated and one feels pain.

Palpate To check the texture, size, and location of parts of the body with the hands.

Paraspinal Adjacent or near to the spinal column.

Pectoral Area of the body on the chest wall going from the shoulder to the underlying breast.

PET scan Positron Emission Tomography. A diagnostic (X-ray) test to preoperatively assess axillary node involvement for staging of breast cancer.

Peristalsis The rhythmic wave of contraction along the intestines, the purpose of which is to propel contents.

pH The scale indicating the level of acidity or alkalinity.

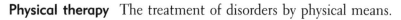

Physical therapy The treatment of disorders by physical means.

Physiologic The workings of the human body.

Physiology The study of the workings of the human body.

Pitting edema An indentation that will take some time to fill back in, caused by pressure to an area of swelling.

Predisposition A latent susceptibility to disease that may be activated under certain conditions.

Pressure stroke The stoke during a massage in a specific direction that applies pressure to the tissue.

Primary lymphedema See Lymphedema, primary.

Prophylactic Guarding from or preventing disease.

Prosthesis An apparatus to replace a part of the body.

Proteins A very large and complex class of amino acids essential to body growth, development, and health.

Proximally Nearest the trunk of the body.

Pycnogenol A bioflavonoid from the bark of the French maritime pine. It is believed to help circulation and to aid in maintaining healthy arteries. The same compound can be found in grape seed.

Quadrant Quarter, section.

Radiation oncology The medical field that treats cancer through radiation.

Radical mastectomy Surgical treatment for breast cancer in which the breast tissue, muscles of the chest wall, a portion of skin, and all the lymph nodes under the arm are removed. Also known as the Halsted radical mastectomy.

Radiotherapy Treatment of disease by means of X-rays or radioactive substances.

Reconstructive surgery Surgery to construct again something that has been removed, such as breast reconstructive surgery after mastectomy.

Rehabilitation To restore to the former state of normal form and function after injury or illness.

Release stroke The stroke during a massage where no pressure is being applied, but in which the hand is moving into a position to prepare for the following stroke that will apply pressure.

Resorption Uptake, as in uptake of fluid from interstitial tissue into venous capillaries.

Secondary lymphedema See Lymphedema, secondary.

Segmental compression Pressure applied sequentially causing the lymphatic fluid to circulate out of the affected limb.

Selenium An element related to sulfur.

Self-massage Massage done by oneself intended to stimulate lymph nodes and to move lymph.

Sentinel node The first lymph node to receive lymphatic drainage from a tumor.

Sentinel node biopsy Surgical procedure in which breast tumor is injected with dye, which is followed along lymphatic vessels to the first node in the axilla. That node is removed and evaluated for cancer. If the node is negative, axillary node dissection can be avoided.

Sequential gradient pump See Vasopneumatic pump.

Shoulder girdle Consisting of shoulder blade, clavicle, upper arm, muscles, and ligaments related to those. The body's support for, and method of, maintaining the shoulder.

Staging Assessing the degree of development of a disease; a stage is a distinct phase in the course of disease; for example, stage I or stage II breast cancer.

Stationary circles In massage, circular motions done in one spot on the body (such as the base of the neck) with the flat tips of the fingers.

Stretch reflex A reflex contraction of a muscle in response to passive stretch.

Subclavian Located under the collarbone.

Supraclacicular Situated above the collarbone.

Systemic Pertaining to or affecting the body as a whole.

Sweep In massage, a gentle pushing in the direction lymph fluid is to flow.

T-Cell A small white blood cell that mainly helps in the immune system.

Tamoxifen A drug used in the treatment of certain types of breast cancer that blocks the action of estrogen.

Theraband A stretchy material (somewhat like rubber) used during certain exercises to increase strength and circulation.

Therapy ball A large, air-filled ball used while exercising. Can assist in building flexibility and strength.

Thoracic duct The main collecting duct of the lymphatic system, receiving lymph from the left side of the head, neck, and chest, the left upper limb, and the entire body beneath the ribs. It is located high in the abdomen and runs up through the thorax (chest).

Thorax The chest area.

Thrombosis The development or presence of a clot or plug in a blood vessel.

Thymocyte A cell of the thymus.

Thymus A gland in the chest behind the sternum and between the lungs. It is a primary central gland of the lymphatic system, housing lymphocytes and macrophages.

T-Lymphocytes Also called "killer cells" because they secrete special compounds that assist B-Lymphocytes in destroying foreign protein.

Uninvolved limb   The limb that does not have lymphedema.

Upper extremity   The arm.

Vascular   Pertaining to vessels.

Vasopneumatic pump   A pump attached to a sleeve that encases the involved arm or leg and segmentally distributes pressure from distal to proximal in order to move lymph out of the limb. Also called a sequential gradient pump.

VEGF-C   Vascular endothelial growth factors. Recent research indicates VEGF-C may, in the future, improve function of the lymphatics after cancer.

Veins   Vessels that transport blood without oxygen back to the heart.

Venous   Having to do with veins.

Venous capillaries   Small veins.

Venous insufficiency   Abnormally low circulation of venous return of blood from the legs to the trunk of the body. Can cause fluid buildup, pain, varicose veins, and ulceration.

Vessel   A small tube in the body that carries fluids such as blood and lymph.

Visualization   The achievement of a visual impression of an object, the picturing of something in one's mind.

Waste products   Debris that is of no use to the system.

Watersheds   The dividing lines between the lymphatic sections of the body, the vertical division being marked by the sternum, the horizontal by the waistline.

Bibliography

Casley-Smith, Judith R., M.D. *Information About Lymphoedema for Patients*, 6th ed. Malvern, Australia: Lymphoedema Association of Australia, 1997.

Casley-Smith, Judith R., M.D. *Modified Treatment for Lymphoedema*, 8th ed. Malvern, Australia: Lymphoedema Association of Australia, 1999.

Glanze, Walter D., ed. *The Signet Mosby Medical Encyclopedia*. New York: Signet/New American Library, 1987.

Hale, Jr., John W. "Lymphatic System." In *Human Anatomy/Physiology*. 6th ed., 716–723. Dubuque, IA: William C. Brown Publishers, 1993.

Beers, Mark H. and Robert Berkow, M.D. *The Merck Manual of Diagnosis and Therapy*. Centennial ed., Whitehouse Station, NJ: Merck Research Laboratories, 1999.

Dorland, W.A. Newman, ed. *Dorland's Illustrated Medical Dictionary*, 24th ed. Philadelphia, PA: W.B. Saunders, 1994.

Thomas, Clayton L., ed. *Taber's Cyclopedic Medical Dictionary*. 18th ed. Philadelphia, PA: F. A. Davis, 1997.

Thiadens, Saskia R. J., R.N. *Lymphedema: An Information Booklet*. 4th ed. San Francisco, CA: National Lymphedema Network, 1996.

Notes

Chapter 1

[1] Saskia R. J. Thiadens, R.N., *Lymphedema: An Information Booklet*, 4th ed. (San Francisco, CA: National Lymphedema Network, 1996).

[2] Jean K. Smith, R.N., M.S., O.C.N., "Oncology Nursing in Lymphedema Management," *Innovations in Breast Cancer Care* 3 (4): 82–87 (September 1998).

[3] M. Grabois, "Breast Cancer Post-Mastectomy Lymphedema," *State of the Art Review, Physical Medicine and Rehabilitation Rev.* 8: 267–277 (1994).

[4] Peter Mortimer, M.D., "The Pathophysiology of Lymphedema," *Cancer Supplement* 83 (12): 2798–2802 (15 December 1998).

[5] Judith R. Casley-Smith, M.D., *Information About Lymphoedema for Patients*, 6th ed. (Malvern, Australia: Lymphoedema Association of Australia, 1997).

[6] Mary Connell, B.S.N., R.N., O.C.N., "Complete Decongestive Therapy," *Innovations in Breast Cancer Care* 3 (4): 93–96 (September 1998).

[7] Dr. James Schwarz, interview with authors, Portland, OR, December 1998.

[8] A. Bollinger et al., "Aplasia of Superficial Lymphatic Capillaries in Hereditary and Connatal Lymphedema (Milroy's Disease)," *Lymphology* 16: 27–30 (1983).

[9] Peter Pressman, M.D., "Surgical Treatment and Lymphedema," *Cancer Supplement* 83 (12): 2782–2787 (15 December 1998).

[10] B. Risher et al., "5-Year Results of a Randomized Clinical Trial Comparing Total Mastectomy and Segmental Mastectomy With or Without Radiation in the Treatment of Breast Cancer," *New England Journal of Medicine* 312: 665–673 (1985).

[11] Armando Giuliano et al, "Sentinel Lymph Node Biopsy for Breast Cancer: Not Yet Standard of Care," *New England Journal of Medicine* 339 (14): 990–995 (October 1998).

[12] Allen G. Meek, M.D., "Breast Radiotherapy and Lymphedema," *Cancer Supplement* 83 (12): 2788–2797(15 December 1998).

[13] Michael Goldman, M.D., interview with authors, Tualatin, OR, 10 April 1998.

[14] Gilbert Lawrence, M.D., "Axillary Dissection in Invasive Breast Cancer," *Oncology* 12 (7): 1011 (July 1998).

Chapter 2

[1] John W. Hale, Jr., "Lymphatic System," in *Human Anatomy/Physiology*, 6th ed. (Dubuque, IA: William C. Brown Publishers, 1993), 716–723.

[2] Kathleen Schmidt Prezbindowski, "Lymphatic System: Non-specific Resistance to Disease and Immunity," in *Principles of Anatomy and Physiology*, 5th ed. (New York: Harper Collins, 1988), 63–69.

[3] Ingrid Kurz, M.D. *Textbook of Dr. Vodder's Manual Lymph Drainage, Volume 2: Therapy*, 2nd ed. (Heidelberg, Germany: Karl F. Haug Publishers, 1989), 73.

[4] "Lymphocyte," in *Signet/Mosby Medical Encyclopedia* (Bergenfield, NJ: Signet New American Library, 1987), 365.

[5] Charles Henderson, "Researchers Discover First Lymphatic Vessel Growth Factor," *Cancer Weekly Plus* 9: 9 (30 June 1997).

[6] Ingrid Kurz, M.D. *Textbook of Dr. Vodder's Manual Lymph Drainage, Volume 2: Therapy*, 2nd ed. (Heidelberg, Germany: Karl F. Haug Publishers, 1989), 43–45.

Chapter 3

[1] Michael Foeldi, M.D., "Treatment of Lymphedema," *Lymphology* 27: 1–5 (1994).

[2] Judith R. Casley-Smith, M.D., "Signs to Be Aware Of for the Onset of Lymphoedema," *Lymphoedema Association of Australia Newsletter* 6 (1996).

[3] *Lymphedema* (Bethesda, MD: National Cancer Institute, 1997), 4. Redistributed by University of Bonn Medical Center, 1997.

[4] Michael J. Brennan, M.D., "Lymphedema After Breast Cancer Surgery," *Journal of Pain and Symptom Management* 7 (2): 112 (1992).

[5] Judith R. Casley-Smith, M.D., "Grades of Lymphoedema," in *Information About Lymphoedema for Patients*, 6th ed. (Malvern, Australia: Lymphoedema Association of Australia, 1997), 5.

[6] "Diagnosis and Treatment of Peripheral Lymphedema, Consensus Document of the International Society of Lymphology Executive Committee," *Lymphology* 28: 113–117 (1995).

Chapter 4

[1] Michael J. Brennan, M.D., "Lymphedema Following the Surgical Treatment of Breast Cancer: A Review of Pathophysiology and Treatment," *Journal of Pain and Symptom Management* 7 (2): 110–116 (1992).

[2] Susan Love, M.D., *Dr. Susan Love's Breast Book*, 2nd ed. (Reading, MA: Addison-Wesley, 1995), 382–385.

[3] Patricia A. Ganz, M.D., "The Quality of Life After Breast Cancer— Solving the Problem of Lymphedema," *The New England Journal of Medicine* 340: 383–385 (4 February 1999).

- Charles L. Loprinzi et al., "Lack of Effect of Coumarin in Women with Lymphedema After Treatment for Breast Cancer," *The New England Journal of Medicine* 340 (5): 346 (4 February 1999).
- [4] Judith R. Casley-Smith, M.D., J. R. Casley-Smith, and Morgan Mason, "Complex Physical Therapy for the Lymphoedematous Arm," *Journal of Hand Surgery* 178 (4): 437–441 (1992).
- [5] "Lymphedema After Cancer," *Health News* 4 (5): 1–2 (April 1998). Source: National Cancer Institute/PDQ Physical Statement, "Prevention and Treatment of Lymphedema After Breast Cancer," *American Journal of Nursing* 4: 34–37 (September 1997)
- [6] Jeanne A. Petrek, M.D., and Melissa Heelan, B.A., "Incidence of Breast Carcinoma–Related Lymphedema," *Cancer Supplement* 83 (12): 2776–2781 (15 December 1998).
- [7] Robert Lerner, M.D., and Jeanne Petrek, M.D., "Diseases of the Breast," in *Lymphedema* (New York: Lippincott-Raven, 1996), 896–903.
- [8] Michael Goldman, M.D., interview with authors, Tualatin, OR, April 10, 1998.
- [9] Judith R. Casley-Smith, M.D., "Information About Lymphoedema for Patients," in *Numbers of Patients with Lymphoedema*, 6th ed. (Malvern, Australia: Lymphoedema Association of Australia, 1997), 8.
- [10] Consensus Document of the International Society of Lymphology Executive Committee, "The Diagnosis and Treatment of Peripheral Lymphedema," *Lymphology* 28: 113–117 (1995).
- [11] Michael Foeldi, M.D., "Treatment of Lymphedema," Lymphology 27 1–5 (1994).

Chapter 6

- [1] H. and G. Wittlinger, *Introduction to Dr. Vodder's Manual Lymph Drainage* (Heidelberg, Germany: Karl F. Haug Publishers, 1986).
- [2] Robert Harris, "An Introduction to Manual Lymph Drainage: The Vodder Method," *Massage Therapy Journal* 31 (1): 55–65 (1992).
- [3] M. Foeldi, M.D., Ethel Foeldi, M.D., and H. Weissleder, M.D., "Conservative Treatment of Lymphoedema of the Limbs," *Angiology, Journal of Vascular Diseases* 36 (3): 171–180 (March 1985).
  - E. Foeldi, M. Foeldi, and L. Clodius, "The Lymphedema Chaos," *Annals of Plastic Surgery* 22 (6): 505–515 (1989).
  - M. Foeldi and L. Clodius, "Therapy for Lymphedema Today," *International Angiology* 3 (2): 207–213 (1984).
- [4] J. R. Casley-Smith, D.Sc., M.B.B.S., M.D., and Judith R. Casley-Smith, M.D., Lymphoedema Association of Australia Home Page, amended, 1997: http://www.lymphoedema.org.au
- [5] Saskia R. J. Thiadens, R.N., National Lymphedema Network circular, 1997.
- [6] Consensus Document of the International Society of Lymphology Executive Committee, "The Diagnosis and Treatment of Peripheral

Lymphedema," *Lymphology* 28: 113–117 (1995).

[7] Robert Lerner, M.D.F.A.C.S., F.I.C.S., "What's New in Lymphedema Therapy in America?" *International Journal of Angiology* 7: 191–196 (1998).

[8] Stanley G. Rockson et al., "Diagnosis and Management of Lymphedema," *Cancer Supplement* 83 (12): 2882–2885 (1998).

Chapter 7

[1] Saskia R. J. Thiadens, R.N., "18 Steps for Preventing Lymphedema," National Lymphedema Network circular (1997).

[2] Kathy LaTour, *The Breast Cancer Companion* (New York: Avon Books, 1993), 380–388.

[3] Saskia R. J. Thiadens, R.N., "Lymphatic Infection: A Constant Fear," National Lymphedema Network circular (1995).

[4] Saskia R. J. Thiadens, R.N., and Mitchelle Tanner, "Lymphedema, Breast Cancer and the Brassiere," *National Lymphedema Network Newsletter* 9 (3): (July 1997).

[5] Carolyn Runowicz, M.D., "Health News," *Lymphedema After Cancer* 4 (5): 1 (April 1998). Source: *New England Journal of Medicine*.

[6] Allen Meek, G.M.D., "Breast Radiotherapy and Lymphedema," *Cancer Supplement* 83 (12): 2788–2795 (15 December 1998).

[7] Peter Mortimer, "Managing Lymphedema," *Clinical and Experimental Dermatology* 20: 98–106 (1995).

• Guenter Klose, "Choices for Chronic Extremity Lymphedema," *Physical Therapy Forum*: 6–8 (November 1991).

• E. Foeldi, M. Foeldi, and L. Clodius, "The Lymphedema Chaos," *Annals of Plastic Surgery* 22 (6): 509 (1989).

• Consensus Document of the International Society of Lymphology Executive Committee, "The Diagnosis and Treatment of Peripheral Lymphedema," *Lymphology* 28: 113–117 (1995).

• Judith R. Casley-Smith, M.D., *Information About Lymphoedema for Patients*, 6th ed. (Malvern, Australia: Lymphoedema Association of Australia, 1997).

[8] Michael J. Brennan, M.D., and Linda Miller, P.T., "Overview of Treatment Options in Management of Lymphedema," *Cancer Supplement* 83 (12): 2821–2827 (15 December 1998).

[9] Linda Miller, B.A., B.S., P.T., "Lymphedema: Unlocking the Doors to Successful Treatment," *Innovations in Oncology Nursing* 10 (3): 53–62 (1994).

[10] Judith R. Casley-Smith, M.D., "Scuba Diving," *Lymphoedema Association of Australia Newsletter* 9 (1995).

[11] Sherry Leved Davis, *Focus on Healing Through Movement and Dance for the Breast Cancer Survivor* (Morro Bay, CA: Enhancement, Inc., 1998).

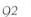

[12] Judith Casley-Smith, Ph.D., M.D., and J. R. Casley-Smith, D. Sc., M.B.B.S., M.D., "Compression Bandages in the Treatment of Lymphoedema," University of Adelaide, 1995. Accessible on the Internet at http://www-med.stanford. ... lymphoedema/bandages.html, 3/97.

[13] Sonja L. Connor, M.S., R.D., and William E. Connor, M.D., chapter 1 in *The New American Diet* (New York: Simon & Schuster, 1989).

[14] Kathy LaTour, *The Breast Cancer Companion* (New York: Avon Books, 1993), 318–329.

[15] U.S. Dept. of Health and Human Services, *Diet, Nutrition and Cancer Prevention: A Guide to Food Choices*, NIH publication no. 87-2878 (Washington, DC: Government Printing Office, 1986).

[16] Sonja L. Connor, M.S., R.D., and William E. Connor, M.D., *The New American Diet Cookbook* (New York: Simon & Schuster, 1997).

[17] Saskia R. J. Thiadens, R.N., "Prevention and Treatment of Lymphedema," *Innovations in Oncology Nursing* 10 (3): 62–63 (1994).

[18] The National College of Naturopathic Medicine, *Guidelines for a Healthy Diet* (Portland, OR: 1996).

[19] Carolyn D. Runowicz, M.D., et al., "Patient Education Pre- and Post-Treatment," *Cancer Supplement* 83 (12): 2880–2881 (15 December 1998).

Chapter 8

[1] Robert Lerner, M.D.F.A.C.S., F.I.C.S., "What's New in Lymphedema Therapy in America?" *International Journal of Angiology* 7: 191–196 (1998).

[2] M. Boris, S.Weindorf, and B. Lasinski, "Persistence of Lymphedema Reduction After Noninvasive Complex Lymphedema Therapy," *Oncology* 11 (1):99–109; discussion 110, 113–4, (January 1997).

[3] Judith R. Casley-Smith, M.D., and John R. Casley-Smith, M.D., "Modern Treatment of Lymphoedema 1. Complex Physical Therapy: The First 200 Australian Limbs," *Australian Journal of Dermatology* 33: 61–68 (1992).

Chapter 9

[1] H. and G. Wittlinger, M.D., *Textbook of Dr. Vodder's Manual Lymph Drainage*, vol. 1, 5th ed., ed. Robert Harris, H.N.D. (Brussels, Belgium: Haug International, 1995).

[2] Michael Foeldi, M.D., "Treatment of Lymphedema," *Lymphology* 27: 1–5 (1994).

 • Joachim E. Zuther, "Understanding Lymphedema," *PT/OT Today* 5 (39): 15–22 (1997).

[3] Renato Kasseroller, M.D., Class Notes from Therapy II and III (Victoria, B.C., Canada: Dr. Vodder School of North America, August 1997).

[4]· H. and G. Wittlinger, M.D., *Textbook of Dr. Vodder's Manual Lymph Drainage*, vol. 1, 5th ed., ed. Robert Harris, H.N.D. (Brussels, Belgium: Haug International, 1995), 74.

[5] H. and G. Wittlinger, M.D., *Textbook of Dr. Vodder's Manual Lymph Drainage*, vol. 1, 5th ed., ed. Robert Harris, H.N.D. (Brussels, Belgium: Haug International, 1995), 73.

[6] Judith R. Casley-Smith, M.D., "Treatment for Lymphoedema of the Arm—The Casley-Smith Method," *Cancer Supplement* 83 (12): 2843–2860 (15 December 1998).

Chapter 10

[1] Judith R. Casley-Smith, M.D., and John R. Casley-Smith, M.D., "Modern Treatment of Lymphoedema I. Complex Physiotherapy: The First 200 Australian Limbs," *Australian Journal of Dermatology* 33: 61–68 (1992).

• H. and G. Wittlinger, M.D., *Textbook of Dr. Vodder's Manual Lymph Drainage*, vol. 1, 5th ed., ed. Robert Harris, H.N.D. (Brussels, Belgium: Haug International, 1995), part B, chapter 1.

Chapter 14

[1] H. and G. Wittlinger, M.D., *Textbook of Dr. Vodder's Manual Lymph Drainage*, vol. 1, 5th ed., ed. Robert Harris, H.N.D. (Brussels, Belgium: Haug International, 1995), 56.

[2] Judith R. Casley-Smith, M.D., "Treatment for Lymphoedema of the Arm—The Casley-Smith Method," *Cancer Supplement*: 83 (12): 2843–2860 (15 December 1998).

[3] Judith R. Casley-Smith, M.D., and J. R. Casley-Smith, D. Sc., M.B.B.S., M.D., "Compression Bandages in the Treatment of Lymphoedema," University of Adelaide, 1995. Accessible on the Internet at http://www-med.stanford. ... lymphoedema/bandages.html, 3/97.

[4] *Legacy Compression Systems*, informal booklet (Seattle, WA: Legacy Systems, 1998).

[5] Judith Casley-Smith, Ph.D., M.D., and J. R. Casley-Smith, D. Sc., M.B.B.S., M.D., "Compression Bandages in the Treatment of Lymphoedema," University of Adelaide, 1995. Accessible on the Internet at http://www-med.stanford. ... lymphoedema/bandages.html, 3/97.

• Renato Kasseroller, M.D., Class Notes from Therapy II and III (Victoria, B.C., Canada: Dr. Vodder School of North America, August 1997).

• Ethel Foeldi, M.D., "Treatment of Lymphedema," *Cancer Supplement* 83 (12): 2833–2834 (15 December 1998).

• Robert Lerner, M.D., F.A.C.S., "Ideal Treatment for Lymphedema," *Massage Therapy Journal*: 37–39 (Winter 1992).

[6] Linda Miller, B.A., B.S., P.T., "An Introduction to the Management of Breast Cancer Lymphedema: An Integrated Approach," from class notes, Anaheim, CA, November 1996.

[7] Judith R. Casley-Smith, M.D., and John R. Casley-Smith, M.D., "Modern Treatment of Lymphoedema 1. Complex Physiotherapy: The First 200 Australian Limbs," *Australian Journal of Dermatology* 33: 63–69 (1992).

Chapter 15

[1] M. Foeldi, M.D., and E. Foeldi, M.D., "Conservative Treatment of Lymphedema of the Limbs," *Angiology* 36: 171–180 (March 1985).

• Judith R. Casley-Smith, M.D., and John R. Casley-Smith, M.D., *Information Booklet of the Lymphoedema Association of Australia* (Adelaide: University of Adelaide, March 1997).

• Joachim E. Zuther, "Understanding Lymphedema," *PT/OT Today* 10 (3): 53–62 (1994).

[2] Linda Miller, B.A., B.S., P.T., "Lymphedema: Unlocking the Doors to Successful Treatment," *Innovations in Oncology Nursing* 10 (3): 53–62 (1994).

[3] Susan Harris and Antoinette Mengers, "Physical Therapist Management of Lymphedema Following Treatment for Breast Cancer: A Central Review of Its Effectiveness," *Physical Therapy* 78 (12): 1302–1311 (1998).

[4] Robert Harris, "An Introduction to Manual Lymph Drainage," *Massage Therapy Journal* 31 (1): 55–66 (1992).

[5] Linda Miller, B.A., B.S., P.T., "An Introduction to the Management of Breast Cancer Lymphedema: An Integrated Approach," from class notes, Anaheim, CA, November 1996.

[6] Robert Lerner M.D., F.A.C.S., "Ideal Treatment for Lymphedema," *Massage Therapy Journal*: 37–39 (Winter 1992).

[7] Judith R. Casley-Smith, M.D., John R. Casley-Smith, R. G. Morgan, and M. R. Mason, "Complex Physical Therapy for the Lymphoedematous Arm," *Journal of Surgery* 178 (4): 437–441 (August 1992).

[8] Peter Mortimer, *Lymphoedema: Advice on Treatment*, 2nd ed. (Beaconsfield, England: Beaconsfield Publishers, 1991), 4–8.

[9] Gottfried Medical Inc., *Information and Instructions for Graduated Pressure Surgical Elastic Supports*, Toledo, OH: manufacturer's pamphlet.

Chapter 17

[1] Michael Foeldi, M.D., "Treatment of Lymphedema," *Lymphology* 27: 1–5 (1994).

[2] E. Foeldi, M. Foeldi, and L. Clodius, "The Lymphedema Chaos," *Annals of Plastic Surgery* 22 (6): 509 (1989).

[3] Judith R. Casley-Smith, M.D., and John R. Casley-Smith, M.D., *Information Booklet of the Lymphoedema Association of Australia* (Adelaide: University of Adelaide, March 1997).

[4] Consensus Document of the International Society of Lymphology Executive Committee, "The Diagnosis and Treatment of Peripheral Lymphedema," *Lymphology* 28: 113–117 (1995).

[5] Guenter Klose, "Treatment Choices for Chronic Extremity Lymphedema," *Physical Therapy Forum* 5 (39): 19–22 (19 November 1991).

Chapter 19

[1] Joan Borysenko, Ph.D., *Minding the Body, Mending the Mind* (New York: Bantam Books, 1988), 62–67.

[2] *Managing Stress and Anxiety Workbook* (Kaiser Permanente, 1996).

Chapter 20

[1] David C. Nieman, *The Exercise-Health Connection* (Champaign, IL: Human Kinetics, 1998), 65–67

[2] James Schwarz, M.D., interview with author, Portland, OR, 1998.

• Allen G. Meek, M.D., "Breast Radiotherapy and Lymphedema," *Cancer Supplement* 83 (12): 2788 (15 December 1998).

[3] Linda Miller, P.T., and Michael Brennan, M.D., "Overviews of Treatment Options and Review of the Current Role and Use of Compression Garments, Intermittent Pumps, and Exercise in the Management of Lymphedema," *Cancer Supplement* 83 (12): 2821–2827 (15 December 1998).

[4] Stanley Rockson, M.D., Linda Miller, P.T., Judith R. Casley-Smith, M.D., Robert Lerner, M.D., et al., "Diagnosis and Management of Lymphedema," *Cancer Supplement* 83 (12): 2882–2885 (15 December 1998).

[5] Michael Alter, *Sport Stretch* (Champaign, IL: Human Kinetics, 1990), 1–25.

[6] Linda Miller, P.T., "Exercise in Management of Breast Cancer–Related Lymphedema," *Innovations in Breast Cancer Care* 3 (4): 101–106 (September 1998).

[7] Kenneth Cooper, M.D., *The Aerobic Program for Total Well-Being*, (New York: M. Evans, 1982), 112.

[8] Charles McGarvey III, "Rehab of the Breast Cancer Patient," in *Physical Therapy for the Cancer Patient* (New York: Churchill Livingston, 1990), 67–84.

[9] Kenneth Cooper, M.D., *The Aerobic Program for Total Well-Being* (New York: M. Evans, 1982), 192–196.

[10] Judith R. Casley-Smith, M.D., "Treatment for Lymphoedema of the Arm—The Casley-Smith Method," *Cancer Supplement*: 83 (12): 2843–2860 (15 December 1998).

[11] Marisa Perdomo, P.T., "Conservative Management of Upper Extremity Lymphedema in Cancer Patients," in *Course Notebook, North American Seminars* (Kirkland, WA: 1998).

Chapter 21

[1] Michael Alter, *Sport Stretch*, (Champaign, IL: Human Kinetics, 1990), 22

[2] Chrissie Gallagher-Mundy, *Essential Guide to Stretching*, (New York: Random House Value Publishing, 1996).

[3] Linda Miller, P.T., "Exercise in Management of Breast Cancer–Related Lymphedema," *Innovations in Breast Cancer Care* 3 (4): (September 1998).

[4] John R. Casley-Smith, M.D., and Judith R. Casley-Smith, M.D., "Aircraft Flights and Scuba Diving," *National Lymphedema Network Newsletter* 7 (3): 8–9 (1995).

[5] James Schwarz, M.D., interview with author, Portland, OR, 1998.

[6] Rosalind Benedet, R.N.C., M.S.N., "Exercise and Diet Benefit Lymphedema Management," *National Lymphedema Network Newsletter* 3 (3):? (July 1991).

[7] David C. Nieman, *The Exercise-Health Connection* (Champaign, IL: Human Kinetics, 1998), 65–67.

Chapter 23

[1] Beverly R. Mirolo, S.R.N., et al., "Psychosocial Benefits of Postmastectomy Lymphedema Therapy," *Cancer Nursing* 18 (3): 197–205 (1995).

[2] Saskia R. J. Thiadens, R.N., "18 Steps to Prevention for Upper Extremities," National Lymphedema Network circular (April 1997).

Chapter 25

[1] Norman Cousins, *Anatomy of an Illness, as Perceived by the Patient: Reflections on Healing and Regeneration* (New York: Bantam Books, 1981), 27–48.

[2] Norman Cousins, *Anatomy of an Illness, as Perceived by the Patient: Reflections on Healing and Regeneration* (New York: Bantam Books, 1981), 48.

[3] Kenneth N. Anderson, *The Signet/Mosby Medical Encyclopedia* (New York: Signet New American Library, 1985), 547.

[4] Mark Golin, "Natural Tranquilizers: Stress Relief That Works Round the Clock," *Prevention* 47 (12): 65 (December 1995).

[5] Philip J. Hilts, "Health Maintenance Organizations Turn to Spiritual Healing," *The New York Times*, 37, December 1995.

[6] Cathy Perlmutter, "Break Free from Fatigue Now and Forever," *Prevention* 48 (12): 102 (December 1996).

[7] Bernie S. Siegel, *Love, Medicine and Miracles* (New York: Harper and Row, 1986), 147–156.

[8] Joan Borysenko, *Minding the Body, Mending the Mind* (New York: Bantam Books, 1987), 36.

[9] Bernie S. Siegel, *Love, Medicine and Miracles* (New York: Harper and Row, 1986), 149.

[10] Bernie S. Siegel, *Love, Medicine and Miracles* (New York: Harper and Row, 1986), 150.

[11] Bernie S. Siegel, *Love, Medicine and Miracles* (New York: Harper and Row, 1986), 156.

Chapter 27

[1] Judith R. Casley-Smith, M.D., "Other Oral Products Which May Be Useful in Place of Coumarin," *Lymphoedema Association of Australia Newsletter*: 2 (1996).

[2] *Nutrition for Today's Living* 57 (7): 34 (July 1995).

[3] Arnold Pike, D.C., "Pycnogenol: A Gift from the Pines," *Let's Live* (reprint), January 1992.

[4] Linda Edwards, "General, Clinical Use of Maritime Pine Pycnogenol," *Fairborne Pycnogenol Monograph* 1: 8 (14 July 1997).

[5] Renato Kasseroller, M.D., correspondence with the authors, 22 July 1997.

[6] J. Anderson, and B. Deskins, "Selenium," in *The Nutrition Bible* (New York: William Morrow, 1995).

[7] Judith R. Casley-Smith, M.D., "What Is Lymphedema?" in *Information About Lymphoedema for Patients*, 6th ed. (May 1997), 3.

[8] Charles L. Loprinzi et al., "Lack of Effect of Coumarin in Women with Lymphedema after Treatment for Breast Cancer," *The New England Journal of Medicine* 340 (5): 346 (4 February 1999).

[9] Diana Brady, "Complementary Holistic Remedies for Lymphedema Treatment," *National Lymphedema Network Newsletter* 8 (3): 8 (1996).

Chapter 29

[1] J. Rovig, M. Miller, and Saskia R. J. Thiadens, "Suggested Guidelines: Questions to Ask When Contacting a Lymphedema Treatment Center," *National Lymphedema Network* special circular (October 1995).

[2] Joan Swirsly, R.N., and Diane Sachett Nannery, "Insurance Issues," in *Coping with Lymphedema* (Garden City Park, NY: Avery Publishing Group), 155–163.

[3] Bill Schuch "New CPT Code Established," *National Lymphedema Network Newsletter* 11 (1): 11 (January-March 1999).

[4] Saskia R. J. Thiadens, R.N., "Current Status of Education and Treatment Resources for Lymphedema," *Cancer Supplement* 83 (12): 2867–2868 (15 December 1998).

Index

THE FEISTY WOMAN'S BREAST CANCER BOOK

by Elaine Ratner. Featured in *The New York Times*

This personal, advice-packed guide helps women navigate the emotional and psychological landscape surrounding breast cancer, and make their own decisions with confidence. Its insight and positive message make this a perfect companion for every feisty woman who wants not only to survive but thrive after breast cancer.

"There are times when a woman needs a wise and level-headed friend, someone kind, savvy and, and caring...[This] book...is just such a friend..." —Rachel Naomi Remen, M.D., author of *Kitchen Table Wisdom*

288 pages ... Paperback $14.95 ... Hardcover $24.95

WOMEN'S CANCERS: How to Prevent Them, How to Treat Them, How to Beat Them

by Kerry A. McGinn, R.N. and Pamela J. Haylock, R.N.

WOMEN'S CANCERS is the first book to focus specifically on the cancers that affect only women—breast, cervical, ovarian, and uterine. It offers the latest information in a clear style and discusses all the issues, from the psychological to the practical, surrounding a cancer diagnosis.

"WOMEN'S CANCERS is fully comprehensive, helpful to patients and healthcare workers alike. Recommended."   —LIBRARY JOURNAL

512 pages ... 68 illus. ... 2nd edition ... Paperback $19.95 ... Hardcover $29.95

RECOVERING FROM BREAST SURGERY: Exercises to Strengthen Your Body and Relieve Pain

by Diana Stumm, P.T.

Speed your recovery from breast surgery, recover mobility, and eliminate pain. In this book, physical therapist Diana Stumm shares what she has learned in her 30 years of working with breast cancer patients. Using clear drawings, she describes a program of specific stretches, massage techniques, and general exercises that form the crucial steps to a full and pain-free recovery from mastectomy, lumpectomy, radiation, reconstruction, and lymphedema.

128 pages ... 25 illus. ... Paperback $11.95

To order books see last page or call (800) 266-5592

CANCER—INCREASING YOUR ODDS FOR SURVIVAL: A Resource Guide for Integrating Mainstream, Alternative and Complementary Therapies *by* David Bognar

Based on the four-part television series hosted by Walter Cronkite, this book provides a comprehensive look at traditional medical treatments for cancer and how these can be supplemented. It explains the basics of cancer and the best actions to take immediately after a diagnosis of cancer. It outlines the various conventional, alternative, and complementary treatments; describes the powerful effect the mind can have on the body and the therapies that strengthen this connection; and explores spiritual healing and issues surrounding death and dying. Includes full-length interviews with leaders in the field of healing, including Joan Borysenko, Stephen Levine, and Bernie Siegel.

352 pages ... Paperback $15.95 ... Hard cover $25.95

CANCER DOESN'T HAVE TO HURT: How to Conquer the Pain Caused by Cancer and Cancer Treatment

by Pamela J. Haylock, R.N., and Carol P. Curtiss, R.N.

Studies have shown that people with cancer benefit by taking control over the treatment of the disease and of their pain. Written with warmth and clarity by two oncology nurses with more than 50 years of experience between them, this guide explains cancer pain, explores the emotional effects on sufferers and caregivers, and shows readers how to manage pain using a combination of medical and natural self-help treatments. Includes a "Self-Care Workbook" section.

192 pages ... 10 illus. ... Paperback $14.95 ... Hard cover $24.95

HOW WOMEN CAN *FINALLY* STOP SMOKING

by Robert C. Klesges, Ph.D., and Margaret DeBon

Strategies for quitting are different for men and women. Women who quit smoking tend to gain more weight, their menstrual cycles and menopause affect the likelihood of success, and their withdrawal symptoms are different. This program is based on the highly successful model at Memphis State University and is authored by pioneers in the field.

192 pages ... 3 illus. ... Paperback ... $11.95

To order books see last page or call (800) 266-5592

MENOPAUSE WITHOUT MEDICINE *Revised 3rd Edition*
by Linda Ojeda, Ph.D.

Linda Ojeda broke new ground when she began her study of nonmedical approaches to menopause more than ten years ago. In this update of her classic book, she discusses natural sources of estrogen; how mood swings are affected by diet and personality; and the newest research on osteoporosis, breast cancer, and heart disease. She thoroughly examines the hormone therapy debate; suggests natural remedies for depression, hot flashes, sexual changes, and skin and hair problems. As seen in *Time* magazine.

352 pages ... 40 illus. ... Paperback $14.95 ... Hardcover $23.95

THE NATURAL ESTROGEN DIET: Healthy Recipes for Perimenopause and Menopause
by Dr. Lana Liew with Linda Ojeda, Ph.D.

Two women's health and nutrition experts offer women almost 100 easy and delicious recipes to naturally increase their level of estrogen. Each recipe includes nutritional information such as the calories, cholesterol, and calcium content. They also provide an overview of how estrogen can be derived from the food we eat, describe which foods are the highest in estrogen content, and offer meal plan ideas.

224 pages ... 25 illus. ... Paperback $13.95

HER HEALTHY HEART: A Woman's Guide to Preventing and Reversing Heart Disease Naturally
by Linda Ojeda, Ph.D.

Heart disease is the #1 killer of American women ages 44 to 65, yet most of the research is done on men. HER HEALTHY HEART fills this gap by addressing the unique aspects of heart disease in women and natural ways to combat it. Dr. Ojeda explains how women can prevent heart disease whether they take hormone replacement therapy (HRT) or not. She also provides information on how women can reduce their risk of heart disease by making changes in diet, increasing physical activity, and managing stress. A 50-item lifestyle questionnaire helps women discover areas to work on.

352 pages ... 7 illus. ... Paperback $14.95 ... Hard cover $24.95

To order books see last page or call (800) 266-5592

ORDER FORM

10% DISCOUNT on orders of $50 or more —
20% DISCOUNT on orders of $150 or more —
30% DISCOUNT on orders of $500 or more —
On cost of books for fully prepaid orders

NAME _____

ADDRESS _____

CITY/STATE _____ ZIP/POSTCODE _____

PHONE _____ COUNTRY (outside of U.S.) _____

TITLE	QTY	PRICE	TOTAL
Lymphedema (paperback)		@ $12.95	
Lymphedema (hard cover)		@ $22.95	

Prices subject to change without notice

Please list other titles below:

		@ $	
		@ $	
		@ $	
		@ $	
		@ $	
		@ $	
		@ $	

Check here to receive our book catalog ❑   FREE

Shipping Costs:
First book: $3.00 by book post ($4.50 by UPS, Priority Mail, or to ship outside the U.S.)
Each additional book: $1.00
For rush orders and bulk shipments call us at (800) 266-5592

TOTAL	_____
Less discount @____%	(_____)
TOTAL COST OF BOOKS	_____
Calif. residents add sales tax	_____
Shipping & handling	_____
TOTAL ENCLOSED	_____

Please pay in U.S. funds only

❑ Check ❑ Money Order ❑ Visa ❑ Mastercard ❑ Discover

Card # _____ Exp. date _____

Signature _____

Complete and mail to:
Hunter House Inc., Publishers
PO Box 2914, Alameda CA 94501-0914
Orders: (800) 266-5592 email: ordering@hunterhouse.com
Phone (510) 865-5282 Fax (510) 865-4295
❑ Check here to receive our book catalog

LYM 11/99